the
hunger
type
diet

the
hunger
type
diet

Discover what drives your hunger,
rebalance your hormones –
and lose weight for good

Lowri Turner

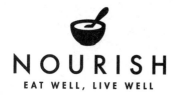

NOURISH

EAT WELL, LIVE WELL

For Griffin, Merlin and Ariel

First published in the USA and Canada in 2015
by Nourish, an imprint of
Watkins Media Limited
19 Cecil Court
London, WC2N 4HE

enquiries@nourishbooks.com

Publisher: Grace Cheetham
Managing Editor: Rebecca Woods
Editor: Jan Cutler
Americanizer: Lee Faber
Designer: Briony Hartley
Production: Uzma Taj

ISBN: 978-1-84899-268-9

10 9 8 7 6 5 4 3 2 1

Typeset in Filosofia
Colour reproduction by PDQ, UK
Printed in Finland

PUBLISHER'S NOTE
While every care has been taken in compiling
the recipes for this book, Watkins Media
Limited, or any other persons who have been
involved in working on this publication,
cannot accept responsibility for any errors
or omissions, inadvertent or not, that may
be found in the recipes or text, nor for any
problems that may arise as a result of preparing
one of these recipes. If you are pregnant or
breastfeeding, or have any special dietary
requirements or medical conditions, it is
advisable to consult a medical professional
before following any of the recipes contained
in this book. Ill or elderly people, babies, young
children, and women who are pregnant or
breastfeeding should avoid recipes containing
raw meat or fish or uncooked eggs.

CAUTION: As with any weight-loss plan,
please consult your doctor before starting
either the 48-hour Hunger Rehab or the 14-Day
Weight Loss Food Plan. Neither is suitable
if you are pregnant, breastfeeding or already
underweight. If you experience any adverse
symptoms, please stop the diet immediately
and consult your doctor.

NOTES ON THE RECIPES
Unless otherwise stated:
• Use large eggs
• Use medium fruit and vegetables
• Use fresh ingredients, including herbs
and spices
• 1 tsp. = 5ml   1 tbsp. = 15ml   1 cup = 240ml

AUTHOR'S ACKNOWLEDGMENTS
Thanks to Borra Garson and Jan Croxson for
helping me to refine the original idea for this
book, and to Grace Cheetham at Nourish for
further guidance and encouragement. Thanks
also to editors Jan Cutler and Rebecca Woods
for knocking the book into shape and to
designers Briony Hartley and Georgina Hewitt
for making it look good.

nourishbooks.com

Contents

Introduction

What is hunger? You may think you know. You may have found that after just one day on most diets you're so hungry that the contents of the cat's bowl can begin to look appetizing, but there are actually different types of hunger. There is genuine physical hunger; the simple, direct hunger, which signals itself with stomach pangs. If the only sort of hunger we responded to was this sort, and we responded to it by sitting down to a nice healthy salad and a piece of grilled chicken, then we would all be slim all the time.

The trouble is, there are other kinds of hunger. And these are the kinds that make you fat. They're the reason you can't resist that creamy dessert, even though you're full already, and why you ignore the diet meal you planned to have for dinner and cook yourself a huge bowl of pasta instead.

Ah, you think, I'm talking about "emotional hunger", the sort where you eat an entire cheesecake when you get dumped. And, yes, to an extent I am. The interplay between emotions and eating is fundamental to the reason why so many people struggle to lose weight. The term "comfort eating" is well known for a reason—so many of us do it.

There is also eating out of boredom or habit, or childhood programming. I have many clients who come to me to help them lose weight who cannot throw food away because they were taught it was wrong to do so. They treat their own body as a trash can instead. I have other clients who "treat" themselves with cake because that's how they were rewarded as a child. Many of us can work our way though a jumbo bag of tortilla chips in front of *America's Got Talent* just because they're there.

Disentangling emotions from food and altering unhealthy patterns set in childhood are vital if you're overweight and want to get the weight off and keep it off. As a hypnotherapist, as well as a nutritionist, I work a lot with so-called behavioral change.

But what this book is really about is the *physical* rather than the *emotional* reasons for weight gain. By this I mean physical imbalances—primarily hormonal—in your body that could be driving your hunger. And, yes, I do realize that this sounds like the oldest excuse in the book (any book): "I'm not overweight because I stuff too many chocolate eclairs. It's my hormones." But those who pooh-pooh the hormone–weight link are actually behind the times.

The obesity epidemic in developed countries is leading to a scientific scramble to try to find a "cure". As part of this research, researchers are looking closely at the biological mechanisms of appetite and weight gain and—surprise, surprise—hormones are proving to play a key role.

In *The Serotonin Revolution: The Low-Carb Diet That Won't Make You Crazy*, I focused on the current new research into three key appetite hormones—serotonin, dopamine and leptin—and showed how you could use this knowledge to help you lose weight. Science doesn't stand still. There are constantly new discoveries, so, as well as the big three, this book looks at new understandings of other hormones—ghrelin, cortisol, gamma-aminobutyric acid (GABA) and others—and how they could be affecting your weight, plus what to do if they are.

WHAT HAVE YOUR HORMONES GOT TO DO WITH IT?

Before men put this book down—don't! We're not just talking about women—men have hormones too, and not just testosterone. They have cortisol, a hormone with a key role in weight gain around your middle, as well as some of the female hormone estrogen. A man's estrogen level should be quite low, but when a man gets "man boobs" it is often a sign of elevated estrogen (a side effect of weight gain in both sexes). The chap with the boobs is becoming feminized. (That should be enough to scare some men into losing weight.)

The body is a series of systems modulated by hormones, which work best in precise ratios to each other. When the ratios become unbalanced, this can result in increased appetite and reduced satiety. A rise in certain hormones can slow down your metabolism or cause more of your food to be stored as fat. Hormonal imbalance can also affect your mood, which can increase appetite and weight. You are not powerless, however. You can alter the balance between hormones just enough to make a difference—to reduce appetite and increase fat burning. All you need to do is find your Hunger Type.

New discoveries into the role of hormones

Research into hormonal imbalance and weight gain began with the discovery of insulin resistance, a condition where your cells cannot respond to the hormone insulin and so your blood sugar and energy levels become unstable. Insulin resistance is known to be a major cause of weight gain and type 2 diabetes. Insulin is a fat-storage hormone, and raised levels should switch off appetite. Those who have insulin resistance produce more and more insulin but they don't stop eating. This leads to weight gain and type 2 diabetes.

Focus has now moved to two other hunger hormones, leptin and ghrelin. It is now believed that you can become resistant to these too. The result is that your natural appetite-signaling system stops working and you never feel truly full, so you keep eating and, yes, you gain weight.

Hunger involves many systems in the body. Other studies are looking at the brain, and specifically the role of neurotransmitters, aka brain hormones, in hunger. Dopamine and serotonin are already well established as being important for weight control, but deficiencies in GABA, an anti-anxiety neurotransmitter, may also increase appetite. Then there is cortisol, the stress hormone. Increased levels have been shown to promote what is known as apple-shaped weight gain—excess weight around the middle. The sex hormones can also play a part: too much estrogen, known as estrogen dominance, or, for women, too little premenstrually or during the menopause, is associated with increased appetite. Too much testosterone in women (which causes polycystic ovarian syndrome—PCOS) or too little in men (causing the andropause) are linked to weight gain.

Is your head spinning yet? Fortunately, you don't need to remember any of this right now, as I'm going to explain it all, and how it applies to you, as we go along. It's worth mentioning now, however, that new hunger hormones are being discovered all the time. Recent additions include neuropeptide Y (NPY), cholecystokinin (CKK), adiponectin, glucagon-like peptide 1 (GLP-1), peptide YY (PYY) and orexins. If this all makes you want to put this book down and go out for a breath of fresh air, good idea. A lack of sunlight can also affect your weight, because it leads to a deficiency in vitamin D, which is associated with depression and increased appetite. Finally we have your DNA. Research is pointing not necessarily to one fat gene but to several.

WHEN THE MESSAGES DON'T GET THROUGH

Hunger is complicated. Far from it being a simple case of a message going from your stomach to your brain to say that the former is empty, so the latter had better tell us to fill it, messages go back and forth constantly. They can be blocked or re-routed or simply not recognized.

Most importantly, I think, all the new appetite research underlines that you are not crazy or weak-willed if you overeat. If you feel hungry all the time, if you can't stop picking or snacking, or if you can't distinguish between emotional and physical hunger and find yourself eating compulsively and/or bingeing, it may be that your natural hunger, or full messaging is simply not working. If you were a house, you'd need rewiring.

That's no reason to give up (so put that family-size bag of salt and vinegar potato chips down now!). There are ways to rebuild the natural hunger message system that will help you lose weight and keep it off. The key is to work out what is driving your eating (your Hunger Type) and then to customize your food and behavior accordingly.

That's what this book is all about. Discover which Hunger Type you are with the quiz, then either do the 48-Hour Hunger Rehab or go straight to your 14-Day Hunger Type Weight Loss Food Plan and start losing weight.

HOW TO USE THIS BOOK

> Even though you may be keen to get stuck into the diet, do take the time to read the next chapter. Understanding the roots of your hunger is empowering. It can allow

you to forgive yourself for past dieting failures and make weight loss in future feel more attainable. The next chapter breaks down hunger into the different Types, and explains in detail what drives them and the different hormonal imbalances that could be driving your hunger. The Hunger Type Quiz follows. Just answer the questions to find out which Hunger Type you are. You may be more than one Type—most people are, so don't worry. Add up your results, then go to the summary of your Type with some specific diet and lifestyle advice to help you lose weight.

> The optional 48-Hour Hunger Rehab follows. This detox is a good way to prepare yourself for a fresh start on your 14-Day Hunger Type Weight Loss Food Plan. It will clear your body of stimulants and processed sugars, which may have caused you cravings in the past. It will also get the weight loss going. But it's tough, which is why it is optional. You can go straight on to your personalized 14-Day Hunger Type Weight Loss Food Plan if you prefer.

> After the Hunger Rehab you can start on your Weight Loss Food Plan. There are 10 plans, each one designed to be perfect for a different Hunger Type. You will know which one is right for you after you complete the Quiz.

> The Hunger Type recipes are the last section of the book. These recipes feature on the Food Plans. The recipes are generally suitable for all of the Hunger Types, but some recipes are more appropriate for particular Types. Either follow your personalized Food Plan to the letter or check below the recipe to see if your Hunger Type symbol is there (see the list opposite). For convenience, I have also put a table of all the recipes starting on page 160 with

cross-references to all the Hunger Types so that you can see at a glance which recipes are right for you.

❯ I have taken the decision not to put any desserts in this book, because I think that if you can get used to not ending your meal with something sweet, in the long term you will keep your weight down. Desserts, on the whole, have no nutritional value. They simply pile on the calories when you are already full—a problem, especially for Hedonistic Hunger Types (see page 48). If you absolutely can't manage without a sweet finish to your meal, or you're at your goal weight, you can save up one of the sweet snacks from the snacks chapter and have that as your dessert.

The Hunger Type symbols

Anxious Hunger

Bored Hunger

Cravings Hunger

Emotional Hunger

Hedonistic Hunger

Never-Full Hunger

PMS Hunger

Stress Hunger

Tired Hunger

Winter-Blues Hunger

40+ Hunger

Right, now let's go back to basics.

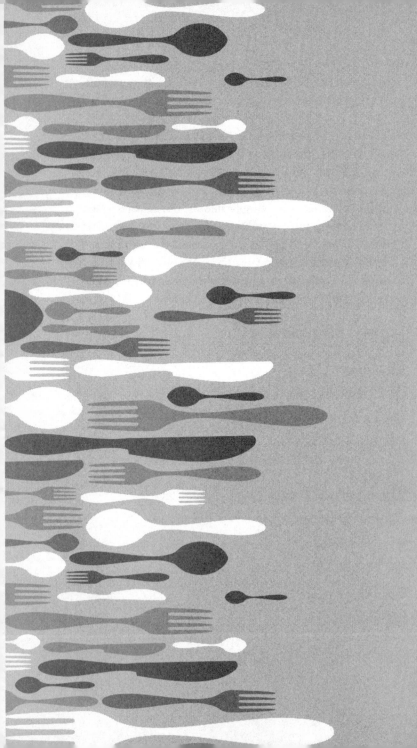

How hunger is supposed to work

There are dozens of hormones and neuropeptides that control appetite, but at its most simple, we can break eating down into three phases: hunger, eating and satiation. Different hormones control different phases, and these are produced in different places in the body; however, the overall control center is the hypothalamus in the brain. Information is sent between the brain, stomach, small intestines and our fat cells to regulate what happens when.

Stage 1—hunger When our stomach is empty, a hormone called ghrelin, which is released by cells in the stomach lining, increases. This sends a message to the brain, making us feel hungry.

Stage 2—eating As we eat, our stomach fills up and the lining starts to stretch. This triggers a reduction in ghrelin production and an increase in another hormone called leptin, which is produced by fat cells. Leptin sends a message to the brain to switch off the appetite. If we eat carbohydrate foods, our blood sugar rises and this triggers the pancreas to release the hormone insulin.

Stage 3—satiety As food moves from the stomach to the small intestine, two hormones, cholecystokinin (CKK) and peptide YY (PYY) are released. These make us feel full and send a message to the brain to stop eating. PYY is stimulated by eating protein-rich foods. Insulin removes the excess sugar from the blood so that it can be burned for energy or stored as fat on our bodies.

Pretty straightforward isn't it? It's a shame it doesn't always work like that.

SO WHY AM I ALWAYS HUNGRY?

There are constant appetite messages going between our brains and our small intestine, as well as others to and from fat cells and the pancreas. Our bodies are simultaneously managing salt balance, detoxification, energy levels, fertility and mood, as well as monitoring external stimuli for any threat resulting in fluctuating stress levels.

If that wasn't enough, when we tip any amount of stimulants or depressants into the mix—such as sugar, caffeine or alcohol—and mess with our natural rhythms of sleep and wakefulness by staying up late to watch TV, we create added challenges for our body to deal with. What's more, many of us live in countries different from our ancestors and eat foods that our digestion wasn't designed for. We live in different ways too. We don't take enough exercise and instead we take medications—the Pill, HRT and antidepressants. No wonder our bodies are confused.

This confusion can cause a whole host of problems with your weight. Let's start with what it can do to the appetite hormones.

WHEN APPETITE HORMONES ATTACK!

As we have seen, there are many, many different appetite hormones. They are designed to help us maintain stasis, or a healthy, stable weight, but sometimes they don't.

Insulin resistance

Insulin is a hormone produced by the pancreas in response to carbohydrate foods being eaten. The carbs break down into sugar during digestion and this sugar makes its way to the blood. Too much sugar is not healthy, so the body releases insulin, which removes the excess blood sugar and sends it to the liver. The liver turns it into glycogen, which is an energy store. Some is kept in the liver and the rest is sent to the muscles. If there's too much sugar, it converts this into fat and stores it on the body.

Insulin resistance occurs when your cells can no longer read the message from insulin. Sugar is not taken out of the blood as it should be, so the pancreas releases more and more insulin, to no effect. Blood sugar and insulin then become dangerously high. Because your cells are not reacting as they should, your hunger switch also gets stuck in the "on" position, so you keep eating and you therefore gain weight.

Leptin resistance

The hormone leptin is released by fat cells whose job it is to tell the brain that you have plenty of fat on your body and you don't need any more, thank you very much, so please stop eating. For people within a healthy weight range, it is a fantastic system for matching appetite to body fat percentage; however, if you gain fat around your middle—also known as central adiposity—you may begin to develop leptin resistance.

The type of "normal" fat that covers you all over in a thin layer beneath your skin is largely benign. You might not like it, but it cushions you from injury and keeps you warm. Visceral fat, on the other hand, is the kind that collects around your midsection (the stuff you can see) and also coats your internal organs, causing things like fatty liver (the stuff you can't)—and it's much more damaging. It is this fat that manufactures the excess leptin which leads to resistance.

The exact mechanism has not yet been agreed upon, but it may be a cry-wolf situation in which the extra fat produces so much extra leptin that your cells just stop listening. The trouble is that, as a result, the appetite stays high and you keep eating and gaining weight.

Ghrelin resistance

Research-wise, ghrelin is the new kid on the block. It works in a push–pull pattern with leptin: leptin switches off hunger; ghrelin switches it on. Ghrelin is released by cells in the stomach lining, which are activated by the stretching that occurs when you fill it up with food. Like insulin and leptin, resistance happens when the message from ghrelin stops working and, even though the stomach is full, appetite is not reduced.

Many overweight people insist that they eat because they feel hungry. Naturally slim people tend to scoff at this and suggest their bigger friends are just greedy; however, ghrelin resistance might provide a physiological explanation for why some bigger people can eat a huge dinner and still feel hungry.

COMFORT EATING

When we feel down, we eat—right? Well, there is the odd person (very odd) who can't bring themselves to so much as nibble on a cookie when they're feeling stressed, but for most of us it's a cue to pick up a large tub of ice cream from the supermarket. Many of us have assumed this is simply because ice cream—or chocolate, or cake—just taste good and they make us feel good. And part of it may be a habit formed in childhood: we fell over and we were given candy, so that starts the stress–sugar link.

There is more going on with comfort eating, though, than just sugary nostalgia. Certain foods have psychoactive properties—that is, they affect the way the brain works. They can make us feel better in a physiological, and not just an emotional, way. A craving for foods such as chocolate or cake is much, much more than just a passing fancy. It could suggest sub-optimal levels of certain key brain hormones, aka neurotransmitters.

Dopamine

The neurotransmitter dopamine does a whole range of things. Crucially, for losing weight, it is involved in learning, memory and decision making, so it helps us stick to a diet. Low levels are associated with starting and not finishing things (bought a gym membership and only gone once, anyone?).

It used to be thought that dopamine itself gave a feeling of pleasure, but now it is believed that it is involved in wanting to feel this pleasure while something else delivers the actual pleasure. Dopamine is important because it drives the pursuit of pleasure, be it through drugs like cocaine, or sex, or … sugar. That doughnut does not give a high of the same magnitude as cocaine, but it acts on the same brain receptors. Ironically, for those trying to lose weight, while high levels of dopamine switch off appetite (cocaine users are not known for frequenting all-you-can-eat buffets), one way to stimulate dopamine production is to eat sugar. This would suggest that a little bit of sugar would be an effective way to lose weight, and indeed "a little bit of what you fancy" is a good maxim for happy weight control, but not everyone can do that. Because dopamine has such a powerful effect, some people may want more—another doughnut, and then some chocolate too, and what about a slice of cake? This is the classic one-cookie-leading-to-a-binge syndrome.

How come the "happy fat person" stereotype is so rarely true (I write as a former fatty myself)? Assuming that weight hasn't been gained by eating loads of green salad, it's more likely to be acquired through a similar amount of cake. And with all that sugar and all that dopamine, you should be feeling fantastic—but you're not.

Leaving aside the guilt that so often comes with not feeling in control of your eating, the problem is that eating a lot of sugary foods over a long time can lead to overstimulation of the dopamine pathway so that it no longer has the required effect. You don't get the good feeling, so you eat more sugar to chase it.

How do you know if dopamine may be driving your overeating? One question you could ask yourself is, "Is there addiction in my family?" Again it's important to say that the notion of "sugar addiction" is controversial, and I certainly wouldn't put it on a par with drug or alcohol addiction. Research suggests, however, that the mechanism is the same, and there may be a genetic element.

Studies indicate that the number of dopamine receptors varies from one individual to another. Those born with few receptors appear to be more prone to addiction of all kinds. This may be because they are trying to overstimulate the ones they have to feel better. If you, or a member of your family, has struggled with overuse of alcohol, drugs, sex or gambling, or with workaholism, it might be a clue. Other relevant behaviors include: being a thrill-seeker (roller coasters, horror movies); changing homes or locations frequently ("doing a geographical"); or switching jobs or relationships regularly. All are suggestive of efforts to stimulate dopamine.

Do the Quiz on pages 94–7 to find out if this is you.

Serotonin

Our very own happy hormone, serotonin, is needed in good levels to reduce appetite and boost mood. Low levels, on the other hand, are associated with depression and often overeating. The drug Ecstasy produces a surge in serotonin. Prozac and other modern antidepressants are actually a class of drugs called selective serotonin reuptake inhibitors (SSRIs). They boost serotonin by keeping what we make circulating in our brains for longer.

You don't have to be clinically depressed to see your appetite affected by low serotonin. We all know that feeling of being down and wanting to treat ourselves to a chocolate bar. After a hard day at work, we may come home and cook a big bowl of pasta. The tranquilizing effect of that chocolate bar or the spaghetti carbonara are not just emotional—they are physical too. They are serotonin highs.

Serotonin is made from an amino acid called tryptophan. We get this from protein foods such as chicken and dairy. But tryptophan is a small molecule that has to compete to jump across the blood–brain barrier. Another hormone, insulin, can help it across, and this, as we have seen, is stimulated by eating sugar. So, without knowing it, many people who use pasta or bread, or sugary foods, to comfort themselves are actually trying to lift their serotonin levels.

It's not just when you're feeling a bit blue that you may crave carbs. Premenstrually, a woman's estrogen levels drop.

Estrogen and serotonin are linked, so mood tends to take a plummet too. Getting sugar cravings just before your period could actually be read as a serotonin craving.

The problem can get worse when a woman goes into her perimenopause, the years post-40 when your production of estrogen declines and you approach the menopause. With estrogen's gentle slide downwards, so serotonin does too, causing sugar cravings to increase. Depression is often cited as a side effect of the menopause, but could this actually be caused by low serotonin? Certainly, I have clients who have never been chocoholics but who get to their mid-forties and can't stop themselves. They can't understand what's happening to them.

The emotional element of the perimenopause and menopause is important. This is an emotional as well as a physical transition; a time when you have to come to terms with not having any more children and/or your older children leaving home. But to see it purely in emotional terms is to verge on misogyny, I think. It's like accusing "older" (how I hate that word) women of being hysterical.

Instead, if you see the forties and fifties as a time of hormonal flux, you can understand why overeating might occur.

GABA

This neurotransmitter is one of the lesser-known ones. Unlike dopamine, which stimulates, GABA inhibits. It is a natural tranquilizer, which helps us deal with stressful and anxious thoughts. It can switch off that "washing machine mind" that afflicts some people when they wake up in the night and go over and over their worries.

We make GABA from the amino acid L-glutamine, which we can make from glutamic acid found in some foods, notably oats and almonds. But we also need plenty of vitamin

B6 to make the conversion. Low levels of GABA may be characterized by a feeling of hyper-vigilance, or constant alertness, even jumpiness. You may bite your nails or lips, or you may find it impossible to sit down to watch a whole movie (two hours of doing nothing!). In terms of what it does to your appetite, though, it can lead to anxious overeating.

All of this is not meant to depress you or make you want to give up, but to arm you with knowledge that you can use to overcome unhealthy overeating so that you can lose weight permanently. Our bodies are making these hormones all the time. Their levels are in a constant state of flux. This means that you can alter the amounts you have by eating the right things, and this can have a fundamental effect on how you feel and behave around food. There may be no one magical "off" switch for hunger, but there are lots of little hormonal switches that you can flick to reduce appetite, reduce fat storage and gain control of your weight.

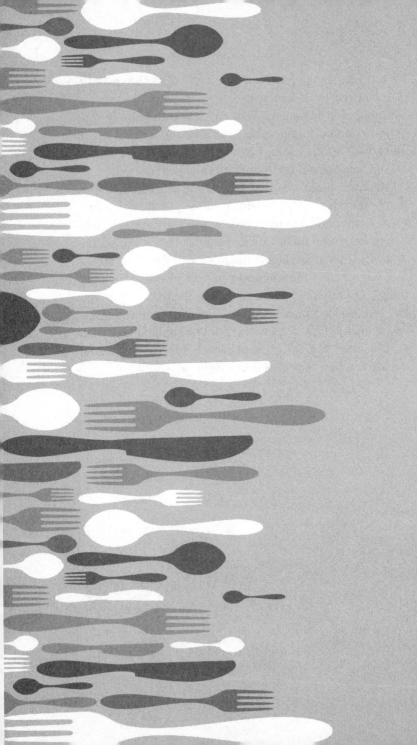

A guide to the different hunger types

If you've read the last chapter, you'll know that there are many different physical mechanisms that can drive hunger—so many, in fact, that it can feel a bit overwhelming. This chapter gets down to the nitty-gritty. It sorts the different appetite and fat-storage mechanisms into 11 easy-to-understand Hunger Types. Each Hunger Type is fully explained, so you can start to work out which one best fits you and find out what to do to start losing weight.

☕ ANXIOUS HUNGER

Do you snack compulsively when you feel anxious or worried? When you are anxious or worried do you make yourself a big meal, eat it and still want to eat more? Do you eat at night, even getting up to eat a snack? If you have Anxious Hunger, you eat to quell fears and worries.

Like Cravings Hunger (see page 33), there is a compulsion to this eating. Those with Anxious Hunger don't eat because they enjoy certain tastes or textures. They eat because they feel they have to. This is not to say that they aren't drawn to particular types of food. In my experience of anxious eaters, they like crunchy foods such as tortilla chips. Perhaps the act of chewing is like a stress ball for the mouth? Soup really doesn't do it.

The volume of food tends to be high with Anxious Hunger, because although you may be eating to ease anxiety, the act of eating is unlikely to solve the problem, so you keep eating to try to get the effect you are after. Also, the act of eating might function as a distraction from the underlying anxiety, so you want to extend this for as long as possible.

What's behind this behavior?
Anxious Hunger is fuelled by the neurotransmitter, or brain hormone, called gamma-aminobutyric acid (GABA). As we have seen, GABA is our very own, naturally occurring Valium. Indeed, GABA binds to the same brain receptors as Valium. If GABA was a person, it would be wearing sandals and a kaftan—its role is to be calming.

GABA is both a neurotransmitter and an amino acid, so we can eat it in our food, but it is a large molecule, too large to cross the blood–brain barrier, so we tend to make it in our bodies instead. It is made from two other smaller amino acids called L-glutamine and L-theanine. The manufacturing process goes via another substance, glutamate (nothing in the brain is simple). Finally, it pops up as GABA.

GABA is the body's most important inhibitory neurotransmitter—that is, it switches stuff off, primarily nerves. In this way it can calm your mind.

This is great if you have an adequate supply, but what if you don't?

What low GABA feels like

The symptoms of GABA deficiency include:

> Anxiety, fear, free-floating anxiety
> Racing thoughts, an inability to relax
> Headaches, fast heartbeat
> IBS
> Carbohydrate cravings

People who are low in GABA often describe themselves as "worriers". If you wake in the middle of the night with worries going around and around in your mind like a washing machine, then it may be that you are low in GABA. And GABA may have a direct role in weight loss.

A type of brain cell called agouti-related protein (AgRP) is known to be crucial to how the brain reads information it gets from the rest of the body about food intake and blood sugar levels, so as to direct appetite and fat storage or burning. New research suggests that GABA may mediate that function. Low GABA could mean that it doesn't work properly.

For those with Anxious Hunger who want to lose weight, however, the most important thing about GABA is its role as a natural tranquilizer, because sub-optimal levels could be at the root of their anxiety and their overeating.

Why do we feel anxious?

Some psychologists believe that there are only two primary human drives—desire and fear. The first is designed to help us reproduce; the second is to keep us alive. The part of the brain where this fear resides is called the limbic system.

The limbic system is common to all mammals and it wraps around the thalamus in the brain. It was named by a French neurologist called Paul Broca in 1878 after the Latin word *limbus*, which means "encircling". The limbic system is responsible for our "fight or flight" response and generates a heightened state of awareness and attention. It's what accounts for the hairs on the back of your neck standing on end when you hear a creak in the night. The limbic system makes us hyper-vigilant in a dangerous situation. It speeds up all our reactions and amplifies information processing from other parts of the brain. We can literally hear a pin drop as we tiptoe downstairs to investigate that creak.

The limbic system is sometimes called the reptilian brain, because it is a primitive structure. It is a throwback to earlier mammalian evolution. Over the course of human evolution, we have developed other more sophisticated parts of the brain, such as the frontal lobe, which expands our emotional range and cognitive storage space. Even so, primitive responses like fear and rage are still modulated by the limbic system.

What's this got to do with your eating? The limbic system can be calmed by GABA, but if you don't have enough of it, you may be permanently in a hyper-vigilant state. The carbohydrate cravings listed as a symptom of low GABA are often an effort to use another calming neurotransmitter, serotonin, to ease anxiety. These carb cravings, however, can lead to weight gain.

There can also be a learned-response element to being a worrier. I have many clients who report panic attacks and/or general anxiety, and when I ask them if their mother or father suffered too, they nod. They have learned to be worried, usually at their mother's quaking knee. If you have Anxious Hunger, some form of psychotherapy or counseling could address the thoughts and beliefs that can contribute to that state.

It's worth mentioning a couple of other brain hormones in connection with the Anxious Hunger Type. Acetylcholine is a neurotransmitter with a stimulant effect. It is vital for the peripheral nervous system, controlling unconscious mechanisms such as heart rate and digestion. It can be the push to GABA's pull, geeing you up while GABA calms you down. Acetylcholine is important for memory and sexual arousal, but too much of it can overexcite the nervous system.

One mineral that affects acetylcholine is magnesium. We can eat this in the form of green vegetables. Magnesium acts to suppress acetylcholine, so calming the nervous system. If you don't get enough magnesium, it can tip the balance in favor of acetylcholine release. The result? Overexcitement of the nervous system. This can be a contributory factor in the anxious feelings fueling the Anxious Hunger Type.

The role of histamine in anxiety

Histamine is another excitatory neurotransmitter. It is released by cells called mast cells, the majority of which are found in places where we could be injured, such as the nose, mouth, feet and gut, as well as in the brain. Histamine is involved in immune response. It helps us react to perceived physical threats from allergens. The streaming eyes and nose of the hay fever sufferer are mediated by histamine, which is why those who have hay fever often take an antihistamine to block its action. What, then, has this got to do with overeating? Histamine can also have a big effect on mental health. There is often a warning on the packets of antihistamine pills: "May cause drowsiness." Users are sometimes advised not to drive while popping the pills. This is because histamine is stimulatory, and suppressing it can have a sedative effect.

High histamine levels can cause anxiety and so be part of the picture for Anxious Hunger Types. Symptoms of high histamine include:

> Excessive thoughts, fast-thinking, OCD
> High achiever, perfectionist
> Shyness, oversensitivity, tearfulness
> Stomach aches, muscle cramps, headaches, migraines
> Susceptible to bouts of adrenal exhaustion

Some scientists even talk about the high-histamine personality, someone who is "go, go, go" all the time. The most obvious clue that you may have high histamine is a tendency toward allergic reactions. If you have hay fever or asthma, sneeze in sunlight or have persistent allergic rhinitis (running or itching of the nose, especially first thing in the morning), you may be a high-histamine personality. Long fingers and toes are also postulated as indicators, although I have my doubts about that. Was ET a high-histamine personality? He had bigger problems, I reckon.

What can you do?
There are certain foods that are believed to raise histamine levels. Animal proteins and dairy foods are top of the high-histamine foods list. Many of the recipes in this book feature exactly these foods, as lean protein can help weight loss. However, there are also plenty of recipes including fish oils and vegetables, which may reduce histamine levels. If you

think that your histamine may be high, it could be worth choosing these pescetarian or vegetarian recipes as the basis for your The Hunger Type Diet.

To sum up then, Anxious Hunger Types who eat to quieten an anxious mind may be low in GABA. They may also have an excess of acetylcholine and too much histamine or be deficient in magnesium, or all of the above. Eating food that is high in glutamic acid, from which glutamine and GABA are made, is a good way to boost GABA. These foods include nuts, lentils and oily fish. There's a reason many people traditionally meet a crisis with a "nice cup of tea" too. Tea contains L-theanine, most important for GABA synthesis.

The 14-Day Anxious Hunger Weight Loss Food Plan is designed to decrease anxiety by boosting GABA, decrease acetylcholine and increase magnesium to reduce overeating and help you to lose weight.

🍚 BORED HUNGER

Do you eat more at home at the weekend than during the week? Do you snack in front of the TV? Do you eat mindlessly? You're at home, you've eaten your dinner, there's nothing on the TV and you're bored, so what do you do? Go out for a nice healthy walk? Read a book? Engage in some improving hobby like constructing a scale model of the Titanic out of matchsticks? Of course not. You eat. You take little tasty morsels out of the fridge, or you scavenge at the back of kitchen drawers and cupboards for the odd stray cookie or slice of cake. In some cases, if you're a mom, you raid the children's bedrooms for an uneaten Easter egg or the candy lurking at the bottom of random party bags (come on, we've all done it).

Bored Hunger has nothing to do with food enjoyment (in contrast to Hedonistic Hunger—see page 48). Often the food you end up eating when you're bored is pretty grim. Because you're trying to pretend you're not actually eating (because you're not physically hungry), you don't cook a balanced meal. Instead, you graze on things that are convenient—potato chips, cookies and other snacks.

Bored Hunger is a compound Hunger Type, as it contains elements of both Cravings Hunger (see page 33) and Emotional Hunger (see page 41).

Boredom—the link to other Hunger Types

If you have Cravings Hunger, you may also eat when you are bored. That feeling of boredom is simply life at a slower pace than you are accustomed to, because you are used to over-stimulating the dopamine pathway in your brain. Dopamine is a stimulatory neurotransmitter (the same one stimulated by cocaine), which gives you a lift. Food can also increase dopamine, so eating becomes not only a way to fill your time and relieve boredom that way, but also, if it is in the form of a high-sugar, high-fat snack like a doughnut, a way to give you a high. If you have Emotional Hunger (see page 41), you may also eat when you are bored. The boredom in this case can be the result of a general listlessness associated with mild depression. Feeling you can't be bothered to do anything and that nothing interests you anyway (except food), suggests low mood as much as boredom. You may then use sugar to increase the antidepressant brain hormone serotonin and so relieve this lackluster feeling.

What can you do?

I haven't designed a specific Bored Hunger Weight Loss Food Plan because I believe it's important to address the underlying issue—Cravings or Emotional Hunger. So you should choose one of those Food Plans instead. Whichever groups you choose, you will also need to think about behavioral change too. It may be that eating because you are bored has also become a habit that you need to conquer. When we keep doing something often enough, it becomes set by our brains as our default. The best way to alter your default is to select an alternative behavior and keep doing it until it becomes the default. If you find yourself eating when you are bored at the weekend, change your location. Go out. If you eat when you are sitting in front of the computer, make yourself a cup of herbal tea to sip instead.

These may sound like pretty feeble suggestions, but if you do anything enough it becomes a habit. The point is just to do something other than eat when you are bored, and if you do it enough, it will become your new habit. In my experience, I would say that it takes a week to bed in a new habit.

Meanwhile, of course, you should be following either the Emotional Hunger Weight Loss Food Plan or the Cravings Hunger Weight Loss Food Plan to keep your hormones and mood stable. And one last thing—boredom is a natural state. Accepting that sometimes you will be bored and doing nothing to alleviate this feeling (especially eating) is another approach you can take.

CRAVINGS HUNGER

Do you feel that there are times when you have to eat something; when you're really driven to it? Are there certain foods that call to you from the kitchen cupboards? Do your efforts to lose weight come unstuck because of a few food favorites that you just can't resist? You may have Cravings

Hunger. Unfortunately, the things you crave are unlikely to be a green salad with no dressing, or a plate of broccoli. Instead, it's chocolate, or ice cream or cake. What's the common denominator of these foods? They are high in fat and off the scale in sugar. The desire for these foods isn't a whim. It isn't that you just happen to pass the office vending machine and have a fleeting thought of how nice a packet of M&M's might be. Those who have Cravings Hunger are ruled by cravings.

Cravings are those yearnings you can't get out of your head. You wake up in the morning thinking about chocolate, you eat your healthy breakfast and you're still thinking about chocolate. You go through all the day thinking the same way until finally you crack at 4 PM and eat a whole bar. And then maybe another one too. "Well," you reason, "I've blown my diet now, so I may as well really blow it." Cravings Hunger is not driven by emotion. Your cravings do not come and go according to how happy or sad you are feeling, or whether your boss has been mean to you or if your partner forgot your anniversary. They are not connected (at least directly) to stress or a lack of sleep, your age or the weather. They exist quite independently of all those and they tend to be constant.

What then drives Cravings Hunger? Yes, of course, high-sugar, high-fat foods taste nice, and that is part of the appeal. But the root of your love for them may not simply be what food technologists call "mouthfeel"—that silky texture of chocolate as it melts on your tongue. The desire for chocolate, cookies, cake, ice cream and so on could be driven by something else: the hormone dopamine.

The dopamine effect

As we have seen, dopamine is a neurotransmitter, or brain hormone, that we all produce in varying quantities. It is connected to feelings of focus, drive, concentration, memory and clear thinking. Those with plenty of dopamine who want to lose weight are focused; they have drive and are able to concentrate on the task in hand—that is, weight loss. They don't forget about their diet the moment they see a cake shop. Symptoms of dopamine deficiency, however, include:

> Lack of motivation and drive (can't get going on things)
> Poor concentration (don't get things finished)
> Tendency toward compulsive behavior and addiction
> Cravings for stimulants (caffeine, sugar)
> Cravings for high-sugar, high-fat foods

Dopamine is found in the frontal lobe of the brain, in the so-called "reward center". There it acts as a kind of traffic policeman, regulating information coming in and going out. This is why good levels promote clear thinking, but to an extent, dopamine is an all-around feel-good drug.

An increase in dopamine can lift your mood, whereas low dopamine can have the opposite effect, and we all know what can happen if you are feeling down—you eat! At its most serious, dopamine-dependent depression (DDD) is characterized by low energy and a feeling that you can't be bothered with anything. It's a pull-the-covers-over-your-head state. DDD is sometimes treated with drugs called monoamine oxidase (MAO) inhibitors. MAO is an enzyme that breaks dopamine down, deactivating it. By reducing the action of MAO, dopamine remains active in the brain for longer, and this has been shown to have an antidepressant effect. Anyone who feels they may have DDD should get advice from their doctor.

How you can boost dopamine
The 14-Day Cravings Hunger Weight Loss Food Plan is designed to boost dopamine production (all your helpful

hunger hormones) in a gentle, natural way, using the food you eat. Here's how.

Dopamine is made from the amino acids L-tyrosine and L-phenylalanine. Amino acids are the building blocks of protein and so, unsurprisingly, we get them from eating protein-rich foods such as meat and dairy. But it is not as simple as you eat some cottage cheese and—hey presto!— your craving for chocolate chip cookies disappears.

Neurotransmitters are part of what scientists call "pathways". A bit like train lines, these can branch off in different directions. The same raw materials, in this case L-tyrosine and L-phenylalanine, can start at one end of the line (as the food you eat) and trundle along, but instead of ending up at the stop marked "dopamine", they continue along the line to another stop called "noradrenaline". Alternatively, L-phenylalanine can bypass dopamine completely and go along a different branch line to make another stimulant called phenylethylamine (PEA) and something else called cholecystokinin (CKK).

PEA has been used successfully to treat atypical depression, so that might help ease some desires to overeat. Similarly, noradrenaline has a stimulatory effect that could lift motivation and focus, both of which can help you lose weight. But if you have genuine Cravings Hunger and your problem is a compulsion to eat high-sugar, high-fat foods, what you may really need is extra dopamine. Unfortunately, you don't get to choose which end product you get from the dopamine pathway.

The negative stress factor

Hormone production may be competitive. This means that when resources are limited, your body has to decide which end product to make. Certain environmental factors can tip this competitive advantage away from dopamine. If, for example, you have a highly stressful job or you are in an unstable relationship, you might be "running on adrenalin"— that is, needing to make a great deal of it. And if you are using all your available resources to produce that, how much is there left to manufacture dopamine?

I said at the beginning of this section that Cravings Hunger exists independently of emotions. Stress, however, has a way of knitting the emotional and the physical together. Stress can cause the release of adrenalin, which could lead both to a more excited state, in which you may be more prone to cravings, and a possible shortage of dopamine, which could also drive cravings.

As a side note, have you heard of that chocolate dessert called Better Than Sex? It is not named accidentally. Sex and chocolate both stimulate dopamine. And increasing dopamine can increase sex drive.

I often see female clients in their forties and fifties who love chocolate but whose sex drive has gone into hibernation. They may be juggling work and school-age children, or caring for elderly parents and experiencing empty-nest syndrome. They may just be in a long marriage in which they feel unappreciated. Menopausal symptoms can also play a role. But boosting dopamine can have a positive result. If you would rather watch TV or eat chocolate than have sex, altering your diet to run along Cravings Hunger Type lines, might help to change things. I'm not saying you'll be re-enacting *9½ Weeks* every night, but it may help.

The pursuit of pleasure

Back to weight loss. An increase in dopamine has been shown to relieve pain, and it boosts feelings of pleasure. It is this last point about pleasure that is really important for Cravings

Hunger. It used to be thought that it was dopamine itself that created these feelings of pleasure, but the current belief is that dopamine drives the pursuit of pleasure, the chase, the desire to feel good. Drugs such as cocaine, crack cocaine, methamphetamine and Ritalin all stimulate the release of dopamine, but so do coffee and cola drinks, and certain behaviors in some people. Sex, gambling, roller coasters or any sort of risky behavior can excite the dopamine pathway. What does it for one person doesn't for another, however, and for some people it's food rather than drugs or sex.

Certainly, the degree of intoxication after eating a doughnut is nowhere near that experienced after a line of cocaine, but there are definite parallels in the experience of "using" junk food.

The addiction link

A recent study from the US investigated the effect on teenagers of looking at pictures of ice cream milkshakes. The teens were shown photos of chocolate milkshakes, then questioned about the foods they craved, and their brains were then scanned. What you would expect to see in response to the photos of the ice cream milkshakes would be a surge of dopamine. But that's not what happened.

All the teens wanted to drink the milkshakes, but those who already routinely ate a lot of ice cream (junk food addicts, in other words) had brains that were less excited by the prospect of eating more. Why? The MRIs showed that their brains displayed signs of dopamine down-regulation— that is, reduced levels of the dopaminic response.

Surely, though, if you eat a lot of fatty, sugary ice cream, you should be swirling in dopamine, shouldn't you? Not necessarily. Addiction is sometimes described as a dulling of the reward circuits, triggered by overuse of a drug. Indeed, one of the hallmarks of drug addiction is that, although dopamine might have been released in large quantities on first trying a drug, once habituated to it, the addict's brain does not release dopamine in the same quantities. The addict then carries on using—trying to chase the initial high. By showing that the regular ice cream eaters had a muted dopamine response, their brain scans demonstrated that they too may have become addicted to the ice cream.

Another US study is interesting for those who have Cravings Hunger, because it not only looked at changes in brain chemistry as a result of a high-sugar, high-fat diet, but it also studied changes in eating behavior. Three groups of rats were fed three different diets. The first got standard rat feed (called chow), and the second was given normal rat feed, plus for one hour a day a smorgasbord of bacon, sausage, icing and chocolate (a high-sugar, high-fat food cocktail). The third group had 24-hour access to this heart attack buffet.

Not surprisingly, the 24-hour buffet group quickly became overweight. The really interesting bit, though, was how determined they became to secure their junk food fix. While access to normal feed was easy, researchers gave the junk food rats mild electric shocks (sorry, animal lovers) when they tried to eat their fatty sugary meals. This did not deter them. They ate compulsively. When their brains were scanned, they too displayed signs of dopamine down-regulation, proving they had become addicted.

What can you do?

The food you eat can make a huge difference to cravings. It can strengthen you against them, plus you can use it to increase your natural levels of dopamine. For this, you need to eat plenty of protein to supply the amino acids from which dopamine is manufactured in the body, as well as some "good" fats (see below for more about these), as these potentiate its effect. The "wiring" in the brain that sends and receives appetite and satiety messages is coated in a covering called the myelin sheath. This is partly made of healthy fats, so you need plenty of them for this to work properly.

You also need a range of vitamins and minerals to act as co-factors for the chemical reactions that go into making dopamine. For the conversion of L-tyrosine and L-phenylalanine into dopamine, you need vitamin B6, iron, magnesium and folic acid. The 14-Day Cravings Hunger Weight Loss Food Plan contains all the raw materials you need to boost dopamine and beat cravings.

Making sense of fats

Fats can be divided into two main groups: saturated and unsaturated. Saturated fats, such as butter and lard, are solid at room temperature. Unsaturated fats, such as olive oil or the fats in oily fish like mackerel and trout, are liquid at room temperature.

It used to be thought that all saturated fat was bad and all unsaturated was good; however, the plot has thickened, so to speak. We now know that there are many different kinds of unsaturated fats. New ones are being discovered all the time. The key to good health now appears to be not just to eat unsaturated fat, but to maintain the correct ratio between the different types.

The most common unsaturated fats are omega-3 (from oily fish), omega-6 (from vegetables and foods like pumpkin and sunflower seeds and their oils) and omega-9 (olive oil). Most of us get a pretty good supply of the omega-6 fats and to a certain extent omega-9, but we are low in omega-3. For Hunger Typers, omega-3 is especially important because it is so well researched as an aid to brain function. Omega-3 has been shown to potentiate brain function, as it improves cell signaling. This is key to getting your Hunger Type hormones to work properly. It is also important for cell signaling in the rest of the body; for example, allowing the sex hormones to do their job effectively.

When it comes to cooking with fat, it is a good weight-control rule of thumb to keep the amount of fat you use to a minimum. Steam, bake or broil, rather than fry. But current research suggests that if you do cook with fat, you're better off using natural fats like butter rather than more manufactured products such as margarines and polyunsaturated oils (vegetable oils), as these may form harmful trans fats. A little olive oil is fine, but the only oil you can really heat to smoke point safely is coconut oil. The upshot? Avoid polyunsaturated margarines (a highly processed product) and cooking oils, as well as packaged food products, which are often high in polyunsaturated fats, and eat oily fish and whole nuts and seeds.

👁 EMOTIONAL HUNGER

Are you a comfort eater? Do you treat yourself with food when you're feeling down? Are bread, pasta, potatoes, rice or wine on your favorite food and drinks list? If you have Emotional Hunger, you use food to manage your emotions. Uncomfortable emotions, such as anger, fear, sadness and guilt are pushed down, or tranquilized, with food, invariably so-called comfort food.

By comfort food, I mean food that is high in carbohydrates. If you crave foods like chocolate, cakes and cookies, and particularly bread, potatoes, pasta and wine, then you may have Emotional Hunger. I know wine is not strictly a food, but it is almost always on the emotional eater's list, because it breaks down into glucose (sugar) in the body, exactly the same as a chocolate brownie or a slice of toast does. Here is my list of the top Emotional Hunger foods and drinks:

> Bread
> Potatoes
> Pasta
> Rice
> Oatmeal
> Wine
> Milk chocolate
> Fruit

What those who have Emotional Hunger may not always be aware of is that even healthy carbs like oatmeal, brown rice and whole-wheat bread break down into sugar. Oh, and fruit. Don't even get someone with Emotional Hunger started on fruit. They practically hyperventilate when I suggest doing without it, which tells a story in itself. If you freak out at the thought of not eating or drinking a particular thing, it's a sign that there is a lot more going on than just liking it. You need it.

Lots of carbs affect your brain

The reason you may need those thick slices of bread, piles of mashed potatoes, bowls of pasta or pieces of fruit is that these foods raise the level of the neurotransmitter, or brain hormone, called serotonin. Serotonin is an inhibitory neurotransmitter, like GABA (see pages 26–7). It can reduce anxiety and aggression, help you feel calm and centered, and reduce appetite (we'll come back to that, obviously).

As we saw earlier, the drug Ecstasy's shiny-happy-people effect is due to a mega-release of serotonin, and when your other half phones you tipsy from the bar and tells you "I weally, weally wuv you …", that could also be a surge of serotonin. A word of caution, though: alcohol lifts serotonin in the short term, although longer term it can actually lower serotonin levels and so cause depression and a rise in appetite.

It is serotonin's antidepressant effect that has excited scientists. Serotonin-dependent depression (SDD) is a form of depression believed to be caused by a chemical imbalance of the brain due to a shortage of serotonin. Unlike reactive depression, which is a reaction to traumatic events and so is best treated with psychotherapy, SDD is commonly treated with drugs called selective serotonin reuptake inhibitors (SSRIs). These keep the serotonin you do have working for longer so that you stay happier for longer. Prozac is the most well-known SSRI.

Now, I'm not suggesting that everyone with Emotional Hunger is clinically depressed. If you feel you are seriously depressed, put down this book and make an appointment to see a doctor. Most of the clients I see who are Emotional Hunger Types are not clinically depressed, but they are down and feel out of control of their eating, especially around sugary, starchy foods.

The link between these foods and serotonin is not a simple one. Serotonin is made from the amino acid L-tryptophan, which we get from eating protein foods. L-tryptophan is converted in the body to 5-hydroxytryptophan (5-HTP). This is then converted again into serotonin. These conversions can only happen if you eat enough protein foods to supply tryptophan (meat and dairy are good sources) and a varied enough diet to give you a range of minerals and vitamins to act as co-factors. You need magnesium, calcium, zinc, iron, folic acid and vitamin B6.

What about sugar?

When amino acids enter the brain, they do so at the so-called blood–brain barrier. It's like waiting at a crosswalk to cross the road. Lots of amino acids are queuing up together, jostling to get across, but only the bigger ones tend to succeed, leaving the smaller ones languishing at the curb.

Tryptophan is a small molecule. What can make the difference for weedy little tryptophan is if he has a bigger, more rufty-tufty amino-acid friend called insulin to help him across. Insulin is stimulated by—ta-dah!—sugar. This is why if you are an emotional eater you may crave sugary foods. You may be unconsciously trying to boost your serotonin levels to lift your mood. Once your serotonin is at a good level, the sugar craving subsides and so does appetite, which is why getting your serotonin up can be so useful in reducing overeating.

Sugar has traditionally been employed as an analgesic (a pain reliever). Babies used to be given sugar water to settle colicky tummies. It was thought that it was the sugar itself that acted as pain medication. Now we know that it is the serotonin effect associated with the insulin release prompted by the sugar that is most likely to achieve that.

It's not just physical pain that serotonin can help, however. Serotonin has a sedative effect on emotional pain too, which is why so many emotional eaters reach for it after a row with their partner, or when their boss has given them a ticking off. What goes up must come down, though, so just as Ecstasy users can suffer a rebound depression as the drug leaves their system, if you eat too much sugar and push your serotonin too high, you can fall off a cliff emotionally as you "come down".

I once went on a weight-loss retreat with a group of overweight sugar addicts. They were the most delightful people when we met while they were all sugared up; however, this being a weight-loss retreat, their sugar supply was cut off. We lived on lentils, nuts and seeds. Days one and two were fine, but by day three, the previously mild-mannered crew had begun to go through sugar, and by extension, serotonin withdrawal. The nice people became demanding and had tantrums. The vegan chef took to hiding in the kitchen.

There may also be a strong element of habit going on with Emotional Hunger. If you were given candy after every grazed knee as a child, you reach adulthood associating sugar with love and care. If you were taken to a candy store at the end of the week as a treat, then you are more likely to want to treat yourself on a Friday evening with a few glasses of wine and a take-out.

Sugar alternatives

One of the central messages of this book is the importance of keeping your blood sugar stable to balance your Hunger Type hormones and reduce cravings. The recipes, therefore, feature very little sugar. Instead, I have used sugar alternatives that give a taste of sweetness with less impact on blood sugar and frequently far fewer calories. →

If you want to make one change to your diet to regain control of your eating, trying these alternative sugars is a really easy first step. They are available from health food stores and increasingly, supermarkets too. Here are your options:

Xylitol Bought as white and granular, xylitol is made from tree sap. It has a low GI and is good for the teeth, although it is a so-called polyol sugar, which can cause stomach ache if eaten to excess. Still, it tastes good and you can bake with it very successfully.

Stevia Bought as white and granular, stevia is made from a leaf. It's very sweet, so usually you find it mixed with other sweeteners, frequently sucralose, so you can use it spoon for spoon like sugar. It has a low GI and is also low in calories. This is the one I use most in the book, because it has the lowest calorie content.

Jaggery Bought as a brown powder, jaggery is made from the bark of a tree and has a slightly caramel taste, which is good in tea, coffee or for baking. It has about half the calories of sugar, but has a low GI and is sweeter, so you use less. It is high in iron too.

Agave syrup Looking like honey, agave syrup is made from a cactus. It has a low GI, but it is a form of fructose, which research is suggesting might be as, or even more, fattening than regular sugar. Nevertheless, it works really well as just a drizzle on pancakes.

Look at your hidden emotions

One of the greatest challenges for people with Emotional Hunger is to strip away meaning from food. Childhood experiences may have resulted in food being weighed down with meaning, both positive and negative. The positive associations of the food you love might be to do with nostalgia—your grandma bought you a particular cake, and eating it reminds you of her. Or it could be negative—your mother banned you from eating chocolate, because she was ashamed of your weight, so you eat it now to spite her.

I am no longer surprised at hearing grown women talk about using food as a weapon against mothers they perceive to be controlling. In the run-up to a family gathering, these women will start to overeat. After a phone call from mom, they will binge. Probe a little deeper and the stories of growing up with a critical and weight-obsessed mom come out. I remember one individual who told me that while at college, she had to call her mother on a weekly basis to report her weight. She was 21.

The low self-esteem that can result from an upbringing like this can in itself feed emotional overeating. Being taught to swallow down "bad" emotions such as anger, sadness, jealousy or fear, rather than express them openly, can make this worse. It can lead to an adulthood where any uncomfortable emotion feels unmanageable unless you sedate yourself with sugar, but this then results in weight gain and yet more uncomfortable feelings.

What can you do?

Of all the types of hunger that cause overeating, Emotional Hunger tends to need the most behavioral change. You may need to challenge deep-rooted feelings and the habit of suppressing these. Emotional Hunger can, however, also be improved at a biochemical level by addressing sub-optimal serotonin levels. Eating in a way that keeps a good, stable level of serotonin in your system by adopting the 14-Day Emotional Hunger Weight Loss Food Plan can really help.

🍲 HEDONISTIC HUNGER

Do you eat a lovely meal, feel quite full, but then see dessert and "find room" for it? Is an open package of cookies an empty package of cookies, as you just have to keep eating until they're finished? You love to cook, and eat at new restaurants—is food your passion?

On the surface, Hedonistic Hunger sounds like fun. In reality, I'm afraid it's not that cheerful, because it causes overeating and weight gain. Hedonistic Hunger is the term coined by scientists to describe the action of eating for pleasure. It could be called greed, and to a certain extent we all do it. We have that one extra slice of really delicious cake, or one extra chocolate or one more spoonful of ice cream, not because we're hungry, but because they taste delicious.

Hedonistic Hunger is a problem when you keep doing it, when it becomes a habit. Because if you get used to indulging yourself in the sorts of foods that give you pleasure—high-calorie ones, usually—you can put on a huge amount of weight and this can cause real health issues: diabetes, heart disease and arthritis.

What's driving Hedonistic Hunger?

There is some research that shows that some people naturally have a more highly developed sense of taste than others. They are natural gourmands who just really, really enjoy food. In my experience seeing many weight-loss clients, Hedonistic

Hunger eaters are often kinaesthetic. This means that they are very sensitive to texture, so they love creamy, melting foods like rich desserts and chocolate. They may also be highly olfactory—in other words, they are turned on by the aroma of foods.

Scientists, though, say that Hedonistic Hunger, just like Cravings Hunger (see page 33), is driven by the hormone dopamine. The difference is that with Hedonistic Hunger you don't really crave one particular food. Your overeating happens because you go after the general good-feeling effect. Eating more of the foods you love stimulates the reward pathway in the brain.

This was demonstrated recently by scientists from the University of Naples. They asked a group of people to eat foods they loved and then they scanned their brains. They subsequently swapped to less delicious foods and scanned the brains again. The researchers discovered that the level of a hormone called 2-arachidonoyl glycerol (2-AG) increased when their volunteers where tucking into food they liked, but not when they were eating food they didn't like so much. The hormone 2-AG activates the dopamine pathway in the brain.

There was another hormone that eating the food they liked switched off, and this was ghrelin. Ghrelin is a hormone produced by cells lining the stomach. As we saw earlier, it is activated by the stretching of the stomach when you have a meal. As your stomach becomes stretched, ghrelin levels usually increase, and this switches off hunger.

In the Italian experiment, ghrelin didn't work, so diners found more space for the foods they loved. On a common-sense level we all know that you can eat a lot more of stuff you like than stuff you don't. But this is the first time a biochemical mechanism for this has been found. For those prone to Hedonistic Hunger, it also suggests a possible solution. Because 2-AG and ghrelin were not affected by less delicious food, avoiding favorite foods may be one way to control hedonistic eating behavior.

What can you do?

I am not suggesting you exist on gruel—the Hunger Type Diet isn't big on gruel. But it might be useful to analyze which are the foods that you can eat more and more of and avoid those, at least for a while. Substituting these foods for ones that do not get the reward center of your brain dancing a fandango could dramatically lessen overeating; for example, I often suggest to chocolate-loving clients that they swap their favorite milk chocolate for dark. They make a face. But I know they are less likely to binge on the dark, because they don't like it as much.

There are other situations that can cause problems for Hedonistic Hunger Types. Variety of food has been shown to stimulate appetite. All-you-can-eat buffets are a traditional area where many people overeat. This is because increasing the number of different dishes available has been shown to stimulate overeating. Eating à la carte or having a take-out are safer options. Switching tastes at the end of a meal can really stimulate Hedonistic Hunger, so if you are going to eat out, avoid dessert.

At home, one idea from the University of Naples research is to eat the food you like most off your plate first. This means that as you move on to less yummy fare, your natural fullness signal in the form of ghrelin works. You begin to feel full and stop eating. Restricting the range of foods at each meal to just three or four might also be useful, as is banning dessert. "Eek!", you say. Lessening the effect of Hedonistic Hunger is one of the main reasons why none of the Hunger Types Food Plans includes any desserts.

🥣 NEVER-FULL HUNGER

Do you eat a meal and never feel really satisfied? Do you eat bigger meals than other people? Do you have a meal and then find yourself craving more food soon afterward?

If you have Never-Full Hunger, you may eat big meals, meals of a size that might have other people going for a lie down afterward, but for you they don't even begin to satisfy. You aren't a snacker. Little and often doesn't do it for you. Instead, you want large volumes of food. This is not to say you don't snack at all.

A really common scenario is for those with Never-Full Hunger to make themselves a large dinner and, because they don't feel sated, almost immediately afterward go on the hunt for more food. It could be something sweet to "finish" the meal, or just something else to chew.

In the past, overweight people who claimed to be permanently hungry were dismissed as greedy. We know now, however, that hormonal changes that occur as a result of gaining weight can actually create the feeling of not being full, and this can cause overeating. You don't feel full, so you eat more and gain weight, but you still don't feel full, so you eat more and gain more weight. And so on and so on.

When the leptin messages don't get through

As I explained at the beginning of this book, appetite and satiety (the feeling of fullness) after eating are controlled by many interconnected hormones. When it comes to Never-Full Hunger, the most important to talk about is leptin.

Here's how it should work. The brain's appetite center, the hypothalamus, can either release neuropeptide Y (NPY), which increases appetite and makes you store fat, or something called pro-opiomelanocortin (POMC), which does the opposite, suppresses appetite and makes you burn fat. Leptin inhibits POMC, so the more leptin you produce, the less hungry you should be.

Leptin is produced by fat cells and it is released in direct proportion to how slim or overweight you are. This is because its role is to keep your weight within a healthy range. The heavier you are, the more leptin you produce and, theoretically at least, the less hungry you should be, so you naturally lose weight.

Leptin works with another hormone called ghrelin, which is released by cells in the lining of the stomach.

The ideal situation is that when it's time to eat, your stomach releases ghrelin, you feel hungry and you have a meal. As you do this, ghrelin levels drop, you feel less hungry and you stop eating. Meanwhile, the amount of leptin released by your fat cells tells your brain either that you are a bit too slim and do need to store some fat, in which case appetite is also stimulated and metabolism slows down, or that you already have enough fat stores, in which case appetite drops and you burn more fat.

That's how it's supposed to work, but if you are overweight you can develop a condition called leptin resistance. Many people have heard of insulin resistance, which can lead to type-2 diabetes, as discussed on page 9. Leptin resistance works in the same way. Your cells can no longer respond as effectively to messages from leptin as they should, so you just keep producing more and more leptin to little or no effect.

Overweight people have been found to have very high levels of circulating leptin. At a point where these levels should be telling the brain to switch off hunger because they already have quite enough weight, thank you very much, the brain is not getting the message. You therefore continue to feel hungry and unsatisfied, and eat.

What might cause leptin resistance?

One reason for leptin resistance might be the type of food and drink you are consuming. Recent research has shown that high-fructose corn syrup (HFCS) blocks the effect of leptin. HFCS, sometimes seen as "glucose-fructose" on food and drink packs, is commonly added to sweet snacks and drinks, aka junk foods. If you are a Never-Full Hunger Type, this is a really strong reason to stay away from these non-foods.

The ghrelin connection

There is another factor that could also be contributing to constant hunger. If you become overweight, you may find that ghrelin no longer works properly either. In one study, overweight people whose ghrelin was checked were found to have very low concentrations, even less than those of a normal weight. Researchers believe that being overweight may increase cell sensitivity to ghrelin so that even a small amount stimulates hunger.

Many people who have Never-Full Hunger have tried multiple diets to try to lose weight. They may even have succeeded for a while. But yo-yo dieting can in itself increase hunger. Dieting has been shown to decrease leptin levels (remember, less leptin means more appetite and a slower metabolism). This means that when you try to lose weight, your body may roll out the leptin big guns to stop you doing it. And even if you do manage to overcome this assault and drop a few pounds, it can slow your metabolism and make you hungrier, so it is much more likely you will regain the weight.

Dieting seems to increase ghrelin levels (remember, more ghrelin means more appetite and a slower metabolism). And, even after you fall off your diet, ghrelin stays elevated. Just like changes to leptin caused by dieting, alteration to ghrelin makes it more likely you will: (a) struggle to lose weight; and (b) struggle even more to keep it off.

It is worth mentioning another important fullness hormone here called peptide YY, also called peptide tyrosine tyrosine or pancreatic peptide YY. It is released 15 minutes after eating and is activated by food filling the stomach. It gives you that satisfied feeling. One of the questions I always ask my weight-loss clients is, "How fast do you eat?" They invariably tell me they eat quickly. If you never feel full, one easy way to counter this is to consciously slow down your eating, to allow peptide YY to kick in. Those from large families may find this more of a struggle, as they have to counter childhood programming that meant if they didn't finish their meals quickly there was no second helping (the fastest eaters always come from families with three or more children).

Peptide YY is released in proportion to the calorie count of the meal you are eating. At first glance this isn't that helpful because you want to eat fewer calories and get more peptide YY to lose weight. But it is also stimulated by meals containing fat and protein. This is one reason why those who eat a junk food diet of high-carbohydrate foods may not feel full. Adding more protein and good fats into your diet may boost peptide YY and help you to feel fuller.

Fiber can help

As fullness of the stomach activates ghrelin, it is also really important for those with Never-Full Hunger to increase the bulk of their meals, without upping the calorie value. The way to do this is to increase fiber.

There are two types of fiber—soluble and insoluble. Insoluble fiber passes through the gut undigested, whereas soluble fiber turns into a gel in the gut, bulking out the stool and improving digestion. Scientists now believe there is actually a third kind of fiber that they have christened resistant starch (RS), which may be especially useful for weight loss. Most starches turn quickly into glucose during digestion, shooting up blood sugar and causing fat storage. RS passes through the digestive tract without turning to glucose.

You can get RS from beans, seeds and whole grains. It is found in especially high amounts in green (unripe) bananas and raw potato, although I'm not suggesting you eat that. Some foods become high in RS once cooked and cooled; for example, beans, bread, potatoes and pasta. The kicker is the last three are also high GI and exactly the ones many people with a weight problem over-eat. The best option, I think, is to aim more for green bananas and beans than bread, potatoes, and pasta. Even then, watch your portion size. RS has been shown to help people feel more full and eat less. RS may also boost metabolism and increase fat burning. It has been shown to improve blood sugar regulation, which is key to helping all Hunger Typers balance their hormones and reduce hunger.

RS starch is actually a form of fermentable carbohydrates; it is fermented by friendly bacteria in the gut. This has another weight-loss benefit. Recent studies have identified a molecule called acetate, which is released when we, or rather the friendly bacteria in our guts, digest a type of RS called inulin. Scientists from Imperial College, London now believe that acetate triggers the release of POMC (see page 51) in the hypothalamus, switching off appetite. The best source of inulin is chicory, but it can also be found in the allium group of vegetables—onions, spring onions and garlic.

As RS ferments, it feeds friendly bacteria in the gut, also called probiotic bacteria. Maintaining a good probiotic level in your body is important for weight loss in a number of other ways too. Probiotics help manufacture energy-giving B vitamins in the body, improving energy release from food and helping you deal with stress. They may improve insulin sensitivity and enhance estrogen metabolism as well, which can reduce fat storage caused by estrogen dominance.

Here comes another hunger hormone (I did warn you there were lots), called cholecystokinin (CKK), which I introduced on page 10. It also helps us to feel full after eating. Boosting that could also help you if you don't feel satisfied after eating. In a recent study comparing the effect of a low-GI diet (one comprised of protein, fats and slow-release carbohydrates) against a high-GI diet (one that has fast-releasing carbohydrates, or lots of fast-release sugars), CKK levels were shown to be higher after the low-GI diet. This means that a low-GI diet could help you feel fuller.

What can you do?

The 14-Day Never-Full Hunger Weight Loss Food Plan is essentially a low-GI diet that has been manipulated to further reduce hormonal imbalance that could be leading to increased appetite and cravings. It is also designed to give a feeling of satiety and fullness by including plenty of lean protein, good fats and vegetables. Look out especially for the dishes marked with the Never-Full Hunger Type symbol.

The glycemic index (GI)

I talk a lot about low GI in this book. For those who aren't familiar with this term, GI stands for glycemic index. It is a measure of how fast carbohydrate foods turn into sugar in the body.

Food with a high GI contains fast-releasing carbs. They give you a quick energy lift, but they then can cause a slump in blood sugar and energy, leading to sugar →

cravings and hunger between meals. This seesaw effect also causes a hormonal cascade that can lead to more of what you eat being stored as fat on your body.

High-GI foods not only include highly processed carbs, such as candy, cakes, cookies and ice cream, but also white rice, pasta and even some sweet fruits and vegetables, such as mangoes, grapes and carrots. Of course, fruit and vegetables have other benefits, notably fiber, which is why there are plenty of vegetables and some fruits on this program. But it's worth bearing in mind that some of the foods you may think of as healthy (for example, fruit salad, butternut squash or dried fruits) may upset blood sugar and cause weight gain.

The Hunger Types Diet is based on low-GI foods. These are carbohydrate foods that release their natural sugars gently, keeping your mood and energy stable and so reducing cravings. Most vegetables are low GI, as are whole grains such as brown rice, quinoa, buckwheat, rye, barley and oats.

Healthy combinations that reduce the GI

Most meals we eat, of course, are not pure carbs, pure protein or pure fat. They are a combination. And this is a very important point about GI. GI only measures sugar, but you can use protein and fat to reduce the GI of a meal, so although a bowl of rice is off the scale GI-wise, as soon as you add some stir-fried chicken (protein) you reduce the GI. Similarly, although an apple is medium GI, by adding some cheese (protein and fat) you take the GI of your snack down. Remember, the benefit of reducing the GI of a meal is that your blood sugar and energy will →

be stabilized, you store less of what you eat as fat and you have fewer sugar cravings. For Hunger Typers, the key is that you feel less hungry between meals.

Adding cheese to an apple is counter-intuitive to serial dieters, many of whom have been taught to regard fat like a vampire avoids garlic. Similarly, putting chicken in your low-cal vegetable soup seems as if it's a step in the wrong direction. But the GI tables, which were developed originally to help diabetics control their blood sugar levels, don't lie.

A baked potato with butter actually has a lower GI than a plain baked potato. A bar of chocolate has a lower GI than a bag of jelly beans. No wonder small children go crazy when you give them an ice cream bar (all sugar/ no fat or protein) on a hot afternoon—the GI sends their blood sugar into orbit.

A word of warning: GI and calories are not the same thing and sensible weight loss means you need to pay attention to both. There is no point in adding great lumps of butter to everything in the mistaken belief that this will lower the GI and help you lose weight. GI is part of the picture, but so are calories in and energy out. Now put down that cream puff!

The perfect balance

The point about low GI is to create balance in your meals. On the Hunger Type Diet you don't eat fruit on its own (high GI); you eat it with yogurt (low GI). You don't even eat brown rice and vegetables (medium GI) on their own; you cook some fish to go with them (low GI). This is a healthy way to lose weight and keep it off.　→

The added twist with the Hunger Types Diet—or strictly speaking the Hunger Types Diets, because there are actually 10 different Food Plans—is it's low GI but with hunger-reducing bells on. Each Food Plan has its basis in low GI, but has been customized to deal with a specific sort of hunger by skewing it toward particular foods that contain those nutrients which have different hunger-reducing effects.

🍵 PMS HUNGER

Do you experience bloating, irritability or other PMS symptoms? Do you have a history of endometriosis, ovarian cysts or another female hormone imbalance? Do you crave chocolate premenstrually? This section is unashamedly aimed at women. Although men do have normal fluctuations in their sex hormone testosterone, this is like the gentle ripple on the surface of the pond when a stone is skipped across it, next to the monthly estrogen–progesterone tsunami that women endure. The rise and fall of these hormones not only controls a woman's fertility, but it also has a huge effect on her mood, her eating and how much of what she eats gets stored as fat—and even *where* it's stored.

The role of estrogen in weight gain

Estrogen is the important hormone for PMS Hunger. One of its roles is to promote fat storage. When its levels start to rise at puberty, this is characterized by girls growing breasts and laying down fat across their hips. Men too have estrogen in their bodies. If they gain weight, their estrogen levels rise.

Those "man boobs" should actually be called "women boobs" as they are the direct result of excess estrogen. They are a feminizing of the male body, which is a scary thought for most men.

But back to women. Premenstrually, many women retain water and feel fatter. They may also eat more, so what is causing this?

The female menstrual cycle can be divided into four phases. Each has its own hormonal profile.

1 **Menstruation** Estrogen and progesterone are low
2 **Follicular** Estrogen peaks
3 **Ovulation** Estrogen begins to drop and progesterone rises
4 **Luteal** Estrogen and progesterone fall dramatically

There are other hormones involved, notably the follicular stimulating hormone (FSH) and luteinizing hormone (LH). There are also multiple endocrine glands, including the ovaries, adrenals, thyroid and pituitary, all of which need to fire off the right hormone at the right time. External factors such as stress, weight loss, over-exercise and poor nutrition can all disrupt a woman's normal cycle.

When it comes to PMS Hunger, it is the final luteal phase that causes the trouble. This is when estrogen and progesterone both drop. Estrogen is linked to the neurotransmitter serotonin (yes, that one again). When estrogen drops, so does serotonin. As already discussed, serotonin has antidepressant and appetite-suppressant effects, so lower serotonin can lead to low mood and overeating. Serotonin depletion can cause cravings, especially for sugar.

But the important thing about PMS hunger and what differentiates it from Emotional Hunger (see page 41) is that it isn't simply low serotonin that is the problem. It is high estrogen. This may seem contradictory. Didn't I just say that it was the monthly drop in estrogen that leads to low serotonin that in turn leads to overeating? Yes, I did. But it is the steepness of that drop that determines the severity of the PMS symptoms and PMS Hunger.

Basically, the higher your estrogen is to begin with, the more roller coaster-ish the drop feels and the more likely you are to be a PMS Hunger Type. One clue that your estrogen may be high can be if you have, or have had, problems like endometriosis or ovarian cysts.

The four PMS types

As ever with hormones, it is actually even more complicated than that. There are actually four types of PMS, each with a slightly different hormonal profile with subtly different effects on your weight and eating. (1) Type A (anxious) with symptoms of anxiety, irritability, jitteriness, pains in joints and muscles, mood swings, self-destructive behavior; (2) Type C (cravings) with symptoms of cravings for sugar, chocolate, pasta, bread or other "comfort" foods, cravings for stimulants such as caffeine in coffee and tea, muscle tremors or heart palpitations, unstable energy; (3) Type H (hyperhydration—water retention) with symptoms of water retention, especially in the breasts, breast tenderness, swelling of hands and feet, bloated stomach, general weight gain; (4) Type D (depression) with symptoms of depression, crying spells, poor short-term memory, trouble sleeping, aggression and paranoia, increased appetite. There is one final type of PMS so serious that it is regarded as a completely separate medical condition: premenstrual dysphoric disorder (PMDD), the most extreme form of Type D PMS. It is marked by extreme depression and even suicidal thoughts. If you think you suffer from this, see your GP immediately.

What causes high levels of estrogen?

The overwhelming cause of PMS and PMS overeating is estrogen dominance. This happens when you have too much estrogen in relation to your other hormones, such as progesterone or testosterone. Your hormones will still go up and down, but in general, the ratio is skewed in the direction of estrogen.

There are two reasons for this; one external and one internal. The external first. We live in an estrogenic world. Our water supply is famously polluted with estrogen from the contraceptive pill. Other substances called xenestrogens, found in plastics, can leak estrogen into the food we eat too.

The internal reason is fat—visceral fat. Fat stored on our legs and bottoms, the traditional places for women to be plumper, is largely harmless. But fat stored around our organs and the crucial muffin-top area, called visceral fat, is not. Fat cells here act like little hormone factories, releasing a steady supply of hormones, including estrogen.

If you put on fat around your middle, you are likely to increase your estrogen levels. By awful irony, estrogen is itself a fat-storage hormone, so more fat means more estrogen means more fat. Even worse, it's not only low estrogen but also high estrogen that can cause you to eat more, so you are caught in a spiral of weight gain. Meanwhile, your PMS gets worse, you overeat because of that and gain even more weight.

The thyroid angle

Another side effect of estrogen dominance can be a depressed thyroid. The thyroid is a tiny gland at the base of the throat that acts like the thermostat on a central-heating system. It sets the "heat" or speed of many body processes, including metabolism. A slower metabolism means more of what you eat may get stored as weight; yet another reason your waistbands may be under strain. Other symptoms to look out for include depression (another reason to overeat), constipation and cold hands and feet.

What can you do?

The answer to PMS Hunger is to reverse estrogen dominance by adopting the 14-Day PMS Hunger Weight Loss Food Plan. This will help balance your sex hormones and so help you lose weight.

🐟 STRESS HUNGER

Have you been through separation, divorce, bereavement or redundancy in the last two years? Do you feel tired at about 6 PM, but then have a "second wind" late at night? Have you gained weight around your midsection? You may think that Anxious Hunger and Stress Hunger are the same thing, but although stress can cause anxiety, the root cause is different. Whereas Anxious Hunger (see page 26) stems from an overstimulation of the limbic system and a possible deficiency of the neurotransmitter GABA, Stress Hunger is marked by an overstimulation of the adrenal glands and a possible excess of another hormone called cortisol.

How do you know if you have Stress Hunger?

> You eat when you're feeling under pressure
> You use food as a coping mechanism in stressful situations and to give yourself a boost of energy and drive
> You're the one who offers to go to the staff lunchroom to pick up chocolate supplies if the team has a tough deadline, or you eat a massive breakfast at the start of a stressful day

Stress Hunger is marked by cravings, especially for sugar and stimulants, but it also sets up a situation where you store more of what you eat as fat. For this reason, Stress Hunger is marked by a characteristic and easily spottable fat distribution pattern. If you eat because you are stressed, you are likely to put weight on across your chest, tummy and back while keeping slim arms and legs. You may also gain weight in your face.

The role of the adrenal glands

At the root of all of this is a pair of organs that sits on top of the kidneys called the adrenal glands. They help your body to mobilize itself in times of stress by releasing a range of excitatory hormones, including testosterone, adrenalin and the stress hormone cortisol. They also help to control salt balance in the body, which is why, when you have been going through a long period of stress and the adrenals are under strain, you may start craving salty foods. If a client says they are craving peanuts or potato chips, for example, I make a mental note "stress".

For Stress Hunger Types, the important hormone to consider is cortisol. It is made in the adrenal glands, but is only released as a result of what is known as the hypothalamic–pituitary axis. It works like this. When a threat is perceived by the brain, a region called the hypothalamus releases corticotropin-releasing hormone. This doesn't in itself stimulate the release of cortisol. Instead, the pituitary gland has to secrete another hormone called adrenocorticotropic hormone (ACTH). It is this that triggers the release of cortisol.

Although, in times of stress, an accompanying shot of adrenalin is responsible for the quick reactions needed to face that threat—it sharpens the senses and speeds up reaction times—it is cortisol that does the stress heavy lifting. Cortisol boosts blood sugar, increases blood pressure and halts non-essential processes such as digestion. It is also a potent anti-inflammatory, should you be injured.

Cortisol is released in a diurnal rhythm—that is, it is high when we wake in the morning and should drop gradually throughout the day. A bit of cortisol feels quite good; however, if you eat because of stress, it is likely that this is due to excess cortisol. This is a syndrome called adrenal stress.

The adrenal stress symptoms

The symptoms of adrenal stress include:

> Tiredness
> Recurrent infections
> Difficulty shaking off these infections
> Poor concentration and jitteriness
> Aches and pains
> Hypoglycemia (low blood sugar with irritability when hungry)
> Low blood pressure and dizziness on first standing up
> Cravings for sugar and stimulants (tea, coffee)
> Flushed, round face and weight gain, particularly around the abdomen
> Easy bruising and purple stretch marks

The reason for the weight gain is largely that Stress Hunger causes cravings for sugar and stimulants. This is because Stress Hunger is underpinned by unstable blood sugar. The desire for sugar and caffeine is an effort to lift blood sugar that has dipped too low. Unfortunately, if you give in to these cravings, you blast your blood sugar upwards and then it plummets again.

This up-and-down blood sugar not only makes your mood unstable (another reason for overeating) but it also exaggerates the stress response in your body you already have, which means more cortisol and more adrenalin. This further promotes the cortisol-related pattern of fat storage — the peanut-on-legs effect.

This stressed fat shape happens because if your body is in a stressed state it seeks to keep a supply of energy that is easy to access—which is near the vital organs. Our organs are stored in our abdomen, hence the layer of fat that can form both around organs such as the liver and under the skin surrounding them.

There is a further problem with adrenal stress. All the hormonal systems in the body are connected, and when you have a problem with your adrenals, this can also affect your thyroid, slowing down metabolism and causing weight gain. Indeed, symptoms of hypothyroid (underactive thyroid) are very similar to those of adrenal stress, and one can be mistaken for the other. The best option is to get your stress levels under control, and this may alleviate any problems with your thyroid.

What can you do?

Apart from going to live on the top of a mountain where you sit cross-legged and hum to yourself gently all day, one of the best ways to recover from adrenal stress, and the eating that is associated with it, is to nourish the adrenals with food and/ or nutritional supplements.

Protein is important, so are essential fats from oily fish, nuts and seeds, and their oils, as they may improve the cell signaling of the hypothalamic–pituitary axis. You can buy what are called adrenal "glandulars". They are potent, and in serious cases of adrenal fatigue I have suggested them, but you may be a bit uncomfortable about eating ground-up animal glands—even if you are not a vegetarian. Fortunately, there is a lot you can do with a combination of stress reduction, exercise and boosting a range of nutrients.

Vitamin C is critical for adrenal function. The highest concentration of vitamin C in your body is in the brain and adrenals. We also excrete more vitamin C in our urine when we are under stress. All the B vitamins help us to deal with stress; in particular pantothenic acid, a deficiency of which has been shown to cause shrinkage of the adrenals. Herbs worth trying include rhodiola, which has been shown to block the stress response in the body.

The 14-Day Stress Hunger Weight Loss Food Plan contains all the raw materials you need to nourish the adrenals and reduce the stress response in your body. This is designed to improve your stress management, reduce stress eating and help you lose weight.

TIRED HUNGER

Do you have trouble getting to sleep, or do you wake in the night? Do you work shifts, travel to different time zones or have a young baby? Do you eat to give yourself energy to get through the day? Those who have Tired Hunger use food for the opposite reason to Anxious eaters (see page 26). They use it to lift themselves up, to give them mental and physical energy. That instant blood sugar spike from a *pain au chocolat* can certainly relieve feelings of exhaustion, but only in the short term. The trouble is, blood sugar will inevitably fall again, then you will feel tired and have to eat more to give you more energy. The result is overeating and weight gain.

The core question to ask yourself is why do you feel tired? One obvious reason can be stress, and if this applies to you, you should be sure to read the Stress Hunger section of this book (see page 63). Tired Hunger, however, is often driven by an imbalance in a crucial sleep hormone called melatonin.

Nurturing your body's natural sleep rhythm

Melatonin is secreted by the pineal gland, located in the hypothalamus region of the brain (a lot goes on there, doesn't it?). The job of melatonin is to send and receive messages to other organs, as well as regulating something called the circadian rhythm. The circadian rhythm is the body's natural 24-hour clock, which sets a regular pattern of changes to things like blood pressure, body temperature and the release of other hormones during the day and night. Most importantly for Tired Hunger, it regulates the sleep–wake cycle.

Melatonin helps us get to sleep and has a key role in deciding how long we sleep for. Levels increase after it gets dark and should peak in the middle of the night, between 11 PM and 3 AM. If you don't have enough natural melatonin, you may have difficulties falling asleep or you might wake during the night and not be able to get back to sleep.

Melatonin is made from the amino acid tryptophan. We eat tryptophan in protein foods like turkey and eggs, and this is then converted in the body into something called 5-hydroxytryptophan (5-HTP). This is then converted to another neurotransmitter, serotonin. This has to be converted once again into melatonin.

There are a lot of steps in the melatonin production process, and none of these conversions can take place without a variety of vitamins and minerals as co-factors, including magnesium, calcium, zinc, iron, vitamin B6 and folic acid. A varied and healthy diet is therefore a vital precursor to good levels of melatonin and good sleep. Eating enough protein to ensure a supply of tryptophan is key, although that might not be enough.

Just like dopamine production, discussed in my section on Cravings Hunger (see page 33), the production of serotonin and melatonin may be competitive—that is, the body has to decide which one to make. If you are low in tryptophan, you might be low in serotonin or melatonin, or both. One of the symptoms of serotonin-dependent depression (SDD) is poor sleep, probably caused by an associated lack of melatonin. Treatment with selective serotonin reuptake inhibitors (SSRIs) such as Prozac can result in drowsiness, probably due to the associated boost in melatonin.

Not all Tired Hunger is the same

There are actually different sorts of disturbed sleep that can result from Tired Hunger. They are:

Advanced sleep phase disorder (ASPD)

> You wake early in the morning (between 2 AM and 5 AM) and feel wide awake, but then feel ready for bed between 6 PM and 9 PM

> It causes overeating, because you use food to push you through that early-evening tiredness.

Delayed sleep phase disorder (DLPD)

> You lie awake tossing and turning into the small hours (4 AM–6 AM typically), then you can't get up in the morning.

> It causes overeating, because you try to jolt yourself awake in the morning by knocking back a strong coffee and/or a high-calorie breakfast.

Free-running sleep patterns

> You get up later and later each day and go to bed later and later (it can also be earlier and earlier) until you are out of sync with normal daylight and darkness.

> It causes overeating, because you may eat multiple meals at odd times of the day.

The importance of darkness

Our circadian rhythm is not exactly 24 hours. It can run at slightly more or slightly less. It is up to melatonin to fine tune the wake–sleep response to keep your 24-hour clock on time. What, then, can upset this delicate mechanism? The principal cause is often light—too much of it.

The conversion of serotonin to melatonin cannot happen without darkness. When the brain senses the onset of night, it directs the conversion of serotonin to melatonin. If you ignore the natural onset of night, switching on lights and TVs and computers, or going clubbing into the small hours, you are altering the natural light–dark rhythm of the day. Your brain doesn't make enough melatonin, and this can stop you sleeping.

It's a real chicken-and-egg scenario. Not going to bed at a decent hour may cause lower melatonin, but low melatonin may mean if you do go to bed you can't sleep.

Researchers say that people are getting an average of two hours less sleep a night today than they then did 50 years ago. In the US, the culture of long working hours means that many are staying at work longer. Others bring work home, have dinner, then open up the laptop or iPad to check emails. Modern technology means we don't get to fully switch off from the stresses of the day.

Even pleasurable interests can keep us up. How many of us now have TVs in our bedrooms (that includes me) or sit up in bed with an iPad checking Facebook? The pressure to "stay connected" is huge. But what does this have to do with weight loss? Put simply, sleep deprivation makes you fat.

The connection between poor sleep and weight gain

There are literally hundreds of scientific papers that have demonstrated a link between lack of sleep and weight gain. Research by the Birmingham Heartlands Hospital in the UK has shown that those who sleep for less than seven hours a night are more likely to become obese.

One reason for this is that lack of sleep appears to increase appetite—we want to eat more when we wake up tired. Subjects in a study who slept less than four hours consumed 900 more calories the next day in snacks alone! At the root of this effect are changes to two crucial hormones. When you are short of sleep, ghrelin, the hormone that stimulates appetite, rises while the hormone leptin, which switches off appetite, falls.

The Tired Hunger Type story doesn't end there. Not only does shortage of shut-eye seem to increase appetite, but it could also change the type of food you choose. In a Swedish study from 2013, 14 men were given $50 each to spend on food on two occasions. The first shopping trip occurred after a full night's sleep, the second after no sleep at all. When shopping after not having slept, the men chose food that was 9 percent more calorific.

When I look at the food diaries of my weight-loss clients, I can spot the nights without them telling me when they've been out tripping the light fantastic and so gone short of sleep. I just have to look at their breakfasts. With the week's diary in front of me, I can see a whole run of good healthy breakfasts (scrambled eggs, yogurt, berries and so on) and then— wham!—it's a big cooked breakfast or a double espresso and a muffin after a night on the tiles. The reason for this sudden loss of self-control may be that tiredness also increases the "reward value" of eating by making certain foods more attractive and increasing our motivation to consume them.

What are these super-tempting foods—lettuce, celery and cantaloupe melon? Of course not. What gets the reward centers of the tired brain lit up like a department store at Christmas is our old friend: high-sugar, high-fat food. The big breakfast and the muffin, plus a hit of caffeine, get the dopamine receptors really jumping.

In a recent brain-imaging study, 23 people enjoyed one night of good sleep and endured another of total sleep deprivation. Then they were shown pictures of junk food. The area of the brain responsible for self-control was less active after sleep deprivation.

There is a theory that self-control is similar to a muscle that can become fatigued. This "limited resource theory" of self-control suggests that after restricted sleep, the strength of your self-control is weakened, making you more likely to have what psychologists term "poor inhibitory control": you see the chocolate croissant and you just can't stop yourself.

Lack of sleep has been shown to literally shut down the brain. Research from Duke-National University in Singapore has demonstrated that sleep deprivation can cause brain function to halt for short periods. MRIs were used to measure blood flow to the brain in people who had been starved of sleep. These people's brains fluctuated from normal function to so-called attention lapses, similar to a power failure that makes the lights on a train briefly go out.

For those who think they have Tired Hunger, there are yet more reasons to get your sleep sorted in order to lose weight. Sleep deprivation has been shown to slow down basal metabolic rate (BMR). This is the rate at which we all burn calories doing normal day-to-day things like sleeping and breathing. The faster your (BMR), the easier it is for you to stay slim.

Muscle loss, weight gain and sleep

Researchers studied 10 people aged between 40 and 50. They all had BMIs that were overweight, but not obese. They were divided into two groups, both of which were put on a diet. The first group were allowed only five and a half hours sleep a night. The second group got eight and a half hours. When they were weighed at the end of the experiment, those who had been allowed less sleep lost 55 percent less weight.

The reason for this might be that sleep deprivation can change your body composition. A study from 2010 looking at the impact of sleep on weight loss found that restricting sleep results in increased muscle loss and decreased fat loss. The more muscle you have on your body, the faster your BMR. If you lose muscle, your metabolism slows down and you are more likely to gain weight.

Sleep deprivation may also slow down the rate at which you burn fat, according to research published in the *American Journal of Clinical Nutrition*. Scientists took a group of men and measured the rate at which they metabolized fat, then they disrupted their sleep with an alarm clock and allowed them an average of only six and a half hours. They then took the measurement again. The men's fat burning was down by a massive 55 percent.

What can you do?

Have you Tired Hunger Typers heard enough (or have you nodded off) yet? The message here is that if you are low in melatonin or you have disrupted or restricted sleep, you gain weight. To reverse that, some of what you need to do is behavioral (go to bed earlier!) but you can also help to boost your natural sleep hormone melatonin with the right diet. Increasing your supply of tryptophan from protein-rich foods is a good start. If you follow the 14-Day Tired

Hunger Weight Loss Food Plan, you will get a good supply of tryptophan and this should improve your melatonin levels and help you to lose weight.

❄ WINTER-BLUES HUNGER

Does cold winter weather make you feel down? Do you eat more comfort foods in winter? Do you put on weight in winter? Winter-Blues Hunger is another variant of Emotional Hunger (see page 41). It is driven by the same hormone — serotonin—although it only happens during winter months and is connected to sunlight. It is well-known that mood can be affected by the time of year. Sufferers of seasonal affective disorder (SAD) get depressed and have low energy in winter. What is less recognized is that they may also eat more.

The symptoms of SAD

Diagnosed SAD is quite rare. Like other forms of depression, it appears to be more common in women, especially aged between 20 and 40. If you think you may be a sufferer, the symptoms to look out for include the following, which should occur between October and March:

> Low mood, often in the mornings
> Lack of energy
> Less get-up-and-go
> Less interest in life
> Being unable to enjoy things
> Irritability
> Seeing other people less
> Less interest in sex

As some of you may have spotted, these symptoms are almost identical to those of clinical depression; however, you can tell if you have SAD rather than non-seasonal depression because: (a) these symptoms appear only in winter; and (b) you eat more. Although those who are clinically (as opposed to mildly) depressed often struggle to eat, SAD sufferers have a tendency to eat more.

The SAD overeating link

Why should this be? Why should winter weather cause increased appetite for some? The answer lies in the amount of daylight available and the effect this has on two key hormones: serotonin and melatonin. I have already talked about these hormones in some detail (see pages 21 and 68), but to recap: serotonin is an endogenous antidepressant — that is, we make it in our own bodies; melatonin is another hormone that triggers sleep.

Serotonin and melatonin are actually part of the same hormonal pathway. Serotonin is converted into melatonin in the body, and this is where the importance of light comes in. Serotonin production is triggered by daylight. Its conversion to melatonin is triggered by darkness. One reason why some people feel so fantastic on a sunny, beachside holiday (apart from the cocktails, of course) may be the boost that the extra daylight in an exotic location gives to serotonin levels.

This is how it should work. As the sun comes up, the light-sensitive layer of cells at the back of your eye, called the retina, convert the light into electrical impulses that travel to a part of the brain called the hypothalamus. This then sends a message to other glands in the body, including the pineal gland, to produce less melatonin. You wake up and start your day.

In winter, however, there is less sunlight around, so melatonin levels can remain higher, giving a permanent feeling of tiredness. With less sunlight, serotonin is also reduced, contributing to feelings of depression and increasing appetite. Cue cravings for comfort food. You don't have to be able to wave a certificate from the doctor reading "I have SAD" to have Winter-Blues Hunger. SAD, like many other conditions, may be regarded as a spectrum disorder—we could all have a bit of it.

Part of Winter-Blues Hunger Type eating could also be convenience. You're not walking around in sleeveless tops and bikinis in February, so you can get away with carrying a bit more weight. Slide on a winter baggy sweater and no one knows how many Mallomars you ate last night.

Essential omega-3 fats and vitamin D

Some SAD sufferers use light therapy to lessen their symptoms; however, nutritional approaches can be really helpful for everyone to reduce the winter desire for comfort food. There is solid research that increasing your omega-3 fats from oily fish like salmon and mackerel, nuts and seeds can help. The people of Iceland have famously low levels of diagnosed SAD and yet they also have dark winters. Researchers think it is their intake of oily fish, which is much higher than our own, that accounts for this.

Omega-3 fats could help Winter-Blues Hunger because they may improve neural messaging. Messages inside the brain are carried along neurones, which have an outer casing like the plastic around electrical wiring, called the myelin sheath. This is partly made of omega-3 fats. A deficiency of these fats can cause messages to "leak" out of the wiring. Boosting these fats has been shown to improve brain function. In particular, this may help potentiate the action of serotonin.

There is another factor to consider if you have Winter-Blues Hunger: vitamin D. Sometimes called the sunshine vitamin, we can make vitamin D by the action of sunlight on our skin—if there is sunlight, of course. In Ibiza in August, you'll be swimming in vitamin D. In Aberdeen in February, hmm, less so. Vitamin D is fat-soluble and we can store it; however, the stores we build up in summer do not usually last through the winter, so there comes a point in January when many people may be deficient in vitamin D. This is important because vitamin D may help weight loss.

In a study, two groups of overweight women were put on a diet. One group was also given vitamin D tablets and they lost more weight. The reason why is not clear, although one explanation could be that vitamin D has an antidepressant effect. One of the jobs of vitamin D is to help the body absorb calcium, which is critical for healthy nerve function. As already discussed, while those who are clinically depressed sometimes eat very little, overeating is a common sign of mild depression.

There are some people who need to watch out more for a potential low vitamin D status. Those who live in northern cities are more likely to be vitamin D deprived, as are those who use sunscreen or people who are darker skinned. Melanin, the pigment that gives skin its colour, blocks the sunlight necessary for vitamin D synthesis.

In developed countries, we are all living more indoor lives, sitting in front of TVs and computers. This means that we are more likely to be low in vitamin D. Researches in the US city of Boston tested people at the end of the summer. Thirty percent of white people, 43 percent of Hispanic people and a huge 84 percent of African–American people were found to be deficient in vitamin D, and the older you get, the less efficient you are at producing vitamin D.

It is estimated that in the UK, three-quarters of all teens and adults are deficient in vitamin D. Are they all also

Winter-Blues eaters? Probably not. But it could be another piece in the puzzle of why obesity is on the rise.

What can you do?

If you think you have Winter-Blues Hunger, you can boost your vitamin D in winter by eating it via oily fish (including mackerel, salmon or trout), eggs, cheese and mushrooms. You can also take supplements, but you need to take the right sort. There are actually two forms of vitamin D in humans. Vitamin D3 (cholecalciferol) is the type made in the body using sunlight. Vitamin D2 (ergocalciferol) is synthesized in plants. Both can be converted into the body into useable vitamin D, although if you're going to supplement, it might be more effective to choose D3.

You also need to increase your serotonin levels, which you can do by eating plenty of tryptophan-containing foods, such as turkey, chicken and eggs, and just a bit of sugar to pop this into the brain. The 14-Day Winter-Blues Hunger Weight Loss Food Plan includes all these foods.

40+ HUNGER

Are you between 40 and 55? Have you started putting on weight, particularly around your middle, and you don't know why? Has your appetite increased or are you now craving specific foods? I debated about whether to put this section in the book. Being over 40 myself, I somewhat bristle at the ageism that suggests there is some sort of cut-off line at 40. Under 40 equals healthy and over 40 equals walker frame. But there are particular hormonal challenges for men and women when they reach what used to be called middle age (another two words I hate, by the way).

For those who may never have had any problems with their weight, suddenly they may start to put on a little, particularly around the tummy. You may go up a bra size or suddenly see an apple shape developing. For many, the reason is a gradual increase in appetite or tendency to comfort eat. One of my clients in her early fifties said to me, "I've never been overweight, but now I just can't seem to stop eating, and I don't know why".

The reason, of course, is 40+ Hunger. There is a similarity for women between 40+ Hunger and PMS Hunger in that they are both connected to estrogen; however, in 40+ Hunger there is another part of the story to consider: the hormone progesterone. Changes to that hormone may be just as vital as those to estrogen. Plus, 40+ Hunger also affects men, via alterations in their testosterone levels.

Some will wonder why I haven't called this section Menopausal Hunger. After all, "the change" is well-known to cause weight gain. But then younger women and all men would have avoided these pages altogether when actually this section can apply to anyone of either gender from age 35 onwards. The hormonal changes that characterize midlife begin a lot sooner than many people think.

To concentrate on the female menopause for a moment, the word "menopause" means the point at which a woman's natural cycle stops. By the time you get to that, however, you may have had many years during which the production of estrogen from your ovaries has been slowing down, causing menopausal symptoms; for example, when women complain of hot flashes, these are caused by a drop in estrogen. Estrogen levels become unstable long before the ovaries actually stop producing it, and it is this instability—one minute it's up, the next it's down—which can unbalance you and cause things like hot flashes.

The beginning of the menopause

The time in your life before your periods stop, but when you tend to experience menopausal symptoms, is called the perimenopause. This can begin at age 35 for some women, but tends to kick in during your mid-forties. Unfortunately, the reduction in estrogen and progesterone production is not a walk down a nice gentle slope, but more like sitting on a seesaw. The genuine menopause, when your hormones settle, can be a relief after the up-and-down excitement of the perimenopause.

How do you know if you are perimenopausal? Symptoms to look out for include:

> Age 35–50
> Still having periods, even if intermittently
> Night sweats and interrupted sleep
> Hot flashes
> Depression
> Low sex drive
> Joint and/or muscle pain
> Hair loss
> Weight gain

The weight gain can be caused by a number of factors. First is the lack of estrogen. In the section on PMS Hunger (see page 59), I discussed what can happen if you have too much estrogen, aka estrogen dominance, and how this causes weight gain. During perimenopause, however, you have the opposite problem: your body is gradually being starved of estrogen.

On one level, you would expect this to mean you lost weight. The trouble is that not only does lower estrogen mean lower serotonin, which can lead to overeating, but your body has a cunning plan to deal with reduced estrogen production from the ovaries, by making it elsewhere—in fat cells. Visceral fat (the fat stored around your organs and midsection) can manufacture estrogen, so less ovarian estrogen can mean more estrogen in fat (adipose estrogen).

If you have 40+ Hunger and a thickening middle, you may be a casualty of your own body's natural inclination to keep its estrogen levels up. Certainly, there is a pretty stubborn biological process at work, as belly fat is notoriously difficult to shift when you're 40 plus. Research suggests that the average person puts on 1–2 pounds every year around their middle from the age of 35–65. Scary!

Midlife symptoms and men

You may have noticed that I said "person" not "woman". That's because this fattening-up process affects men as well as women. The andropause is the name for the midlife hormonal shift that affects men, although some doctors now prefer the term partial androgen deficiency in the aging male (PADAM). Whatever you call it, it is estimated to cause problems for up to 10 million men in the US each year. Symptoms sound remarkably similar to those experienced by women at the perimenopause:

> Tiredness
> Loss of sex drive
> Depression
> Poor memory and clouded thought
> Disturbed sleep
> Weight gain

Some men can even get hot flashes and night sweats. For men with 40+ Hunger, the reason they may begin to gain weight is declining production of male hormones, principally testosterone. The production of testosterone falls gradually from age 40 onwards. Other hormones are also affected, including growth hormone, insulin-like growth factor (IGF-1), parathyroid hormone and malenocyte-stimulating hormone (MSH). Dihydroepiandrosterone (DHEA) is another androgen, produced in the adrenal glands, and it too declines with age.

One in five of men over 50 are now thought to have what has been christened testosterone deficiency syndrome. But many more will see their waist size increase. The reason is that as androgens fall, so the balance with other hormones, such as estrogen, is altered, making its effect more pronounced. Men can then suffer the same problems as estrogen-dominant women in that they gain weight around their middles. This fat manufactures more estrogen and they gain more weight. And around and around it goes.

What can compound things for men is that the drop in testosterone they may experience removes a natural weight-loss advantage that younger men have over women. Men naturally carry more muscle than women, and as muscle is more metabolically active than fat, this speeds up their metabolism. It is the muscular advantage that makes it both easier for young men to maintain a healthy weight and lose weight when they want to. Men over 40 are losing muscle mass all the time, which changes their shape and makes it more likely they will gain weight. Andropause-associated depression can also lead to eating more and certainly being less active, so that is another reason you may put on a few pounds.

Men can have their testosterone levels checked, but a word of caution. Simply getting a figure for total testosterone isn't that useful. Here's why. Testosterone is carried around the body in your blood bound to a protein, almost like riding piggyback. Sixty to 70 percent of the testosterone in a man's body is bound to something called sex hormone-binding globulin (SHBG). It is not active in this form and the link between the testosterone and SHBG has to be broken for it to have any effect on you.

Older men tend to produce more SHBG, meaning more of the testosterone they produce is inactive. There is another protein that also "binds" to testosterone as well, called albumen. It too makes the testosterone inactive. Only about 2 percent of a man's total testosterone is actually free and active. To get an accurate picture of your testosterone level you need a "free testosterone test". These are expensive and quite difficult to get.

What can you do?

For men who have low testosterone, one option is androgen therapy, otherwise known as injecting yourself with testosterone. This is a controversial treatment, available only through a doctor's prescription. Some scientists are concerned about a possible rise in the risk of prostate cancer.

Women are also offered hormone replacement therapy (HRT) to smooth out the menopausal ride, either estrogen or estrogen and progesterone together. And female HRT is also controversial. For some it is a godsend, although personally I am queasy at the thought of women being medicated for life, first with the Pill and then with HRT. Studies come and go linking HRT to raised risks of cancer and then seeming to disprove this.

Theoretically, HRT should help with 40+ Hunger because estrogen may relieve serotonin-driven sugar cravings; however, many women report weight gain on HRT. Doctors have consistently disputed this, saying it is just water retention. But then they have always said that about the Pill, and yet talk to anyone who has been on that and we all know you do gain weight. Whether HRT-related weight gain is water retention or not, you feel fatter. As the phrase goes, if it walks like a duck and quacks like a duck, it is a duck. The point is, you can't do up the zip on your jeans. My gut instinct is that unless you are put on HRT for medical reasons, it is not helpful for 40+ Hunger, particularly if you are already overweight. Yes, you may not be producing estrogen from your ovaries, but you could be producing plenty from your visceral fat stores, and this could actually result in estrogen dominance. Many women over 40 also have underactive thyroids, which slow down the metabolism. Increasing estrogen could further depress the thyroid, leading to more weight gain.

Right at the beginning of this section I said that 40+ Hunger differed from PMS Hunger in that it was caused not just by estrogen but by progesterone too. There is an argument that the appetite-stimulating, fat-storing effects of estrogen dominance for older women are compounded by the fall in progesterone that otherwise could offset the estrogenic effect. Remember, both these hormones drop perimenopausally, but visceral fat makes more estrogen, but not more progesterone, so the balance tips in favor of estrogen.

In the US there has been a lot of interest in progesterone with a boom in over-the-counter progesterone creams, as an alternative to conventional estrogen or estrogen–progesterone-combined HRT therapy. Not only is progesterone therapy believed to relieve menopausal symptoms but it is also being touted as a way to avoid middle-aged spread.

Doctors in the UK caution against the use of self-administered progesterone creams. They are available only on prescription in the UK. It should also be said that progesterone does not have the same well-documented bone-strengthening benefits of estrogen, so those with a family history of osteoporosis who want to use HRT would probably do better to choose a combined therapy, including estrogen. That said, for women with 40+ Hunger, eating foods that promote progesterone synthesis may be a good idea to reduce weight. There aren't many foods that do that, but egg yolk and dairy foods boost progesterone. Supporting the thyroid is also essential, as this is so often depressed by estrogen dominance.

For men and women who have 40+ Hunger, correcting hormonal imbalance is key. Keeping your blood sugar stable, reducing stimulants and eating enough protein and healthy fats to potentiate helpful hunger hormones by adopting the 14-Day 40+ Hunger Weight Loss Food Plan can really help.

What should you drink?

Keeping your blood sugar, energy and mood stable is essential. A large latte on the way to work or half a bottle of Chardonnay when you get home will unbalance your system, setting off cravings and causing weight gain. Alcohol can weaken resistance and lead to late-night bingeing and comfort eating to deal with a hangover.

No alcohol is allowed on any Hunger Type Food Plan. I've lost count of the number of people who've told me they're doing Diet X "with wine"—it doesn't work.

You should also limit caffeinated tea and coffee to no more than one per day, with food (to slow down the caffeine hit). Fruit juice, fruit drinks and carbonated sweetened drinks should be avoided. Drink water (up to 4 cups per day), herbal teas and decaf coffee.

AND FINALLY, DO YOU HAVE FAT GENES?

Were you overweight as a child? Do you come from a "fat" family? Are you always on a diet? This isn't strictly a Hunger Type, because the cause is not a specific hormone imbalance, but rather a quirk of your DNA. Still, I'm including it here because, for those who struggle to lose weight, it may be both cheering to know that it might not be your fault and, most importantly, there are things you can do to overcome a "bad hand", genetically speaking.

I once interviewed a doctor who had spent 30 years developing treatment programs for overweight children. He said to me, "I never see an overweight child without an overweight parent." This is not parent bashing. The truth is that fat almost always runs in families. This is partly an issue of family culture. Parents, even the most well-intentioned, who themselves eat large portions or consume a lot of high-sugar, high-fat foods are more likely to feed their children that way.

There is a concept called "fat contagion" that scientists have studied, which has shown that the size of the people with whom you spend time has an effect on your own weight. Being from a "bigger" family may give you "permission" to be overweight. It normalizes it. It can also normalize the behavior that could lead you to becoming overweight—not exercising, treating yourself with food, eating the "wrong" foods; however, there is increasing research that there can also be genetic reasons for weight gain. Those who struggle to lose weight may literally have "fat DNA".

The set point theory

The idea that some are destined to be fatter than others has been around since the 1950s when the Set Point Theory was first postulated. This theory says that we all have a set point for our body weight, which our body will fight to maintain. If your set point is low, that's great, but if it is high, then even if you diet, your body will slow down your metabolism to try to keep that high set point. We now know that the chemical basis for this is the action of hunger hormones such as leptin.

The genetic influence on weight

A new theory, known as "thrifty gene syndrome", emerged a decade or so ago which says that some people are genetically programmed to store more of what they eat as fat. More recently, research on gut flora, which help us release energy from food and so have a vital role in fat storage or burning, has suggested that some people's gut flora works more efficiently to help fat storage than others. These people have a "thrifty" gene.

In truth, there are hundreds of genes with a role to play in body weight. A US study by the University of Louisville looked at the data of 57,000 people and found a link between five genes and increased waist-hip ratio (WHR). WHR is a much more accurate measurement of overweight and obesity than the traditional body mass index (BMI), because increased WHR actually measures central adiposity: the apple-shaped weight gain that is associated with unhealthy weight gain rather than just being heavier, which can be skewed by completely healthy muscle mass.

The US researchers discovered three new genes associated with greater WHR in men and two in women. One of the genes linked to elevated WHR in women is called SHC1. It appears to activate insulin receptors and increase the growth of fat cells. In experiments, mice without this genetic variant were leaner than those with it.

A further study, from Cambridge University in the UK, identified mutations to another gene that could cause weight gain. Over 2,000 people were studied, including those who were overweight. People who had been severely obese since childhood were shown to have alterations to a gene called KSR2. These people had an increased appetite as children and a lower metabolic rate as adults. Experiments showed that the KSR2 gene makes cells less able to mobilize fatty acids for fuel – that is, to burn these calories rather than store them—leading to weight gain.

In Israel, a family containing 13 morbidly obese members was compared to 31 other families with normal BMIs. The obese family were found to have a mutated gene that may result in excessive weight gain. The altered gene in question produces a protein called CEP19. Scientists altered this same gene in mice and they went on to be twice the size of normal mice, with twice the level of body fat. They were also diabetic, ate more and moved less than other mice.

It is already established that having a gene called FTO predisposes you to being fatter, but researchers from the University of London in the UK now think they know why. They tested two groups of normal-weight men. One group was regarded as "high risk" in that they had a double dose of FTO (both their parents were FTOs). Both groups were given a meal and then their levels of ghrelin checked. Ghrelin, which you will remember stimulates hunger, did not drop after eating as much in the FTO group as in the "normal" group. It also began to climb more quickly after eating in the FTO group.

Low dopamine and its effect on genes

The action of dopamine, the hormone that drives addiction and is also at the root of the Cravings Hunger Type (see page 33), appears to have an important genetic component. Faulty gene coding resulting in low levels of dopamine receptors in the brain, called DRD2 receptors (D2 for short), could play a role in a preference for sugar and fat. Brain scans of the adult children of alcoholic parents have revealed low levels of these crucial D2 receptors.

Experiments on rats have further revealed a link between this trait and overeating. Rats whose brains have been modified to artificially reduce the number of D2 receptors have been shown to eat insatiably. Plus, the brain scans of these rats have displayed dopaminic down-regulation, indicative of sugar addiction.

In another study from the Oregon Research Institute, using photos of ice cream, a classic high-sugar, high-fat dopamine-boosting combo, two groups of slim people had their brains scanned. Those who had obese parents experienced a bigger surge of dopamine when they looked at the ice cream. The suggestion is that, despite being slim themselves, those with obese parents had inherited a different dopamine response, further fuel for the overeating DNA argument.

PCOS and weight problems

There is one more hormonal condition in which DNA may play a role. Polycystic ovarian syndrome (PCOS) is a blood sugar disorder in women of childbearing age that results in excess testosterone. It also causes weight gain and seems to run in families. It is also associated with stress. Some of the symptoms are:

> Infertility or difficulty getting pregnant
> Skin breakouts along the jaw line or on the chest or back
> Excess hair on the face, especially the chin, also in some cases on the stomach
> Poor blood sugar regulation resulting in hypoglycemia (dizziness and irritability when hungry)

> Muscular frame; good at sport
> Feeling dizzy upon first standing up
> Sugar and/or a craving for stimulants
> Weight gain

PCOS is often not diagnosed until you have trouble getting pregnant. It doesn't mean you can't have a baby, but it may make it more difficult. One clue can be from female relatives on your mother's side who have also had infertility problems or struggled with their weight. Those who are not trying to have a baby may be offered the Pill to suppress symptoms, but you can manage it effectively with a low-GI diet (see page 56) and regular exercise.

What can you do?

All the Hunger Type Food Plans are based around the low-GI principles that are most helpful for PCOS sufferers. Getting your weight down, learning to deal with stress better and taking exercise can reduce, or even eliminate, symptoms.

For non-PCOS sufferers who think you may have "bad" DNA and are ready to throw in the gym towel, don't. There are things you can do to overcome a genetic predisposition to put on weight. Exercise has been shown to overcome your set point, probably by potentiating the action of leptin. Exercise also improves insulin sensitivity, particularly if you exercise after eating, thus leading to less fat storage.

Other research is revealing that the type of food you eat can influence the addictive response. Interestingly, the same rats that gorged themselves on junk food did not do the same when fed only standard rat feed. They also did not display addictive dopaminic down-regulation. It was the junk food that appeared to switch on the overeating and addiction mechanisms. This is not to suggest that you eat the human equivalent of standard rat feed, which sounds pretty grim. But avoiding high-sugar, high-fat foods may switch off the gene that makes you gain weight.

DNA in itself does not guarantee that you will be a certain way. It is a genetic predisposition plus an environmental trigger that does that. You can control those triggers to some extent. You can decide to eat properly and exercise. You can keep an eye on your portion sizes and reduce your stress levels. You can adopt one of the Hunger Type Food Plans, which will help you get your weight down and keep it there.

> Balance your blood sugar by avoiding stimulants and refined sugar, and building your diet around lean protein, healthy fats and whole grains to lessen inherited compulsive behaviors.

> Establish a regular routine of meals, and keep a food diary (see page 177). Chaotic eating leads to overeating and weight gain. Take control of your food: pack your lunch and cook your meals at home.

> Change the family culture. If you live with an overweight partner or overweight family members, get them onside. Discuss changes that you can all make, such as throwing out the cookies, walking the dog or going to the gym.

> Take a probiotic tablet daily. Thrifty gene syndrome is connected to low levels of friendly bacteria in the gut, which help to release energy from food. Boost yours.

> Exercise daily. A combination of cardio and resistance exercise has been shown to overcome your body's set point.

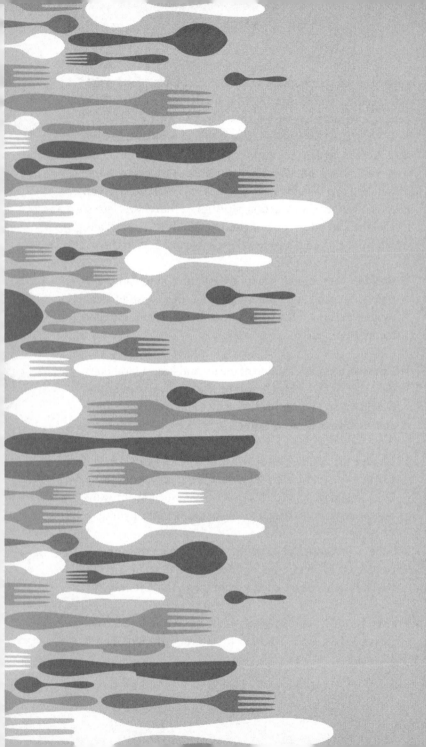

What hunger type are you?

Take the Quiz to find out which Hunger Type is the most appropriate for you, then go to the relevant summary section for some diet and lifestyle tips. Remember, you may be more than one Hunger Type, which would mean that you can combine one or more Food Plans for your Hunger Type Diet. When you move on from your 14-day plan, I recommend that you aim for as many of those recipes marked for your hunger type, or types, as possible.

The optional 48-Hour Hunger Rehab is your next step after the Quiz to get you ready to start your personalized Hunger Type Diet.

Quiz

Please read the following questions, answering yes or no to each, then go to Find Your Hunger Type to find out what your answers mean.

1 My mother was a "worrier" and so am I.   YES / NO

2 I suffer from headaches, indigestion, fast heartbeat,
   IBS, panic attacks or insomnia.   YES / NO

3 I eat quickly, sometimes not really realizing
   I am doing it until the food is gone.   YES / NO

4 Evenings and weekends are my danger
   time for overeating.   YES / NO

5 I eat in front of the computer, TV or in the car.   YES / NO

6 I am a snacker or grazer.   YES / NO

7 I am an "all or nothing" person.   YES / NO

8 An open package of cookies is an empty packet
   of cookies. I cannot just eat one.   YES / NO

9 Someone in my family has a history of problems
   with alcohol, drugs, gambling, sex, computer
   games, or was/is a heavy smoker, or changed
   homes or locations frequently.   YES / NO

10 When I am upset, I eat to make myself
   feel better.   YES / NO

11 My favorite foods are bread, pasta, rice
   and potatoes.   YES / NO

12 I know I can relax when it gets to "wine o'clock". YES / NO

13 Dessert is my favorite part of a meal. YES / NO

14 I love cooking and eating out. I consider myself a foodie. YES / NO

15 Diet food is boring, so I find it hard to stick to a weight-loss plan in the long term. YES / NO

16 There is no "off" button for me with food. I never feel full. YES / NO

17 I am more than a stone overweight. YES / NO

18 I eat bigger meals than other people. YES / NO

19 Usually, I eat well, but in the days before my period, I binge on sugar. YES / NO

20 I have a history of endometriosis and/or ovarian cysts. YES / NO

21 I have always been curvy, with a D-cup bra size or larger. YES / NO

22 I "run" on tea/coffee or diet cola. YES / NO

23 Although I feel tired by about 6 PM, I get a second wind around 10 PM and can stay up late. YES / NO

24 My favorite snacks are potato chips, peanuts or other salty/highly flavored foods. YES / NO

25 Sleep is a problem for me. I either can't get to sleep or I wake in the night. YES / NO

26 My job involves foreign travel, shifts and/or I have a young baby. YES / NO

27 Food gives me energy to get through the day. YES / NO

28 I tend to put on weight in the winter. YES / NO

29 Sunshine cheers me up and I feel happiest on a beach holiday. YES / NO

30 When it's dark outside, all I want to do is stay in bed. YES / NO

31 I am over 40. YES / NO

32 I have never had to worry about my weight, but now I can't stop eating. YES / NO

33 My doctor has suggested that I take HRT (women) or statins (men). YES / NO

FIND YOUR HUNGER TYPE

The questions are divided into categories. If you answered yes to two or more questions in the question groups below, you will find the Hunger Type category that relates to you.

Eek! My answers say I'm more than one hunger type! If you answered yes to two or more questions in several question categories, you have more than one type of hunger. This is very common. All you need to do is read the results for each different Hunger Type you scored highly in, then choose the 14-Day Emotional Hunger Type Weight Loss Food Plan, as this is most suitable for compound Hunger Types. You can choose to customize it by including recipes from other Hunger Types you scored highly in, if you like. Just look at the table at the back of the book to select the right ones.

1–3   You are an Anxious Hunger Type (go to page 98)

4–6   You are a Bored Hunger Type (go to page 104)

7–9   You are a Cravings Hunger Type (go to page 106)

10–12   You are an Emotional Hunger Type (go to page 112)

13–15   You are a Hedonistic Hunger Type (go to page 118)

16–18   You are a Never-Full Hunger Type (go to page 124)

19–21   You are a PMS Hunger Type (go to page 130)

22–24   You are a Stress Hunger Type (go to page 136)

25–27   You are a Tired Hunger Type (go to page 142)

28–30   You are a Winter-Blues Hunger Type (go to page 148)

31–33   You are a 40+ Hunger Type (go to page 154)

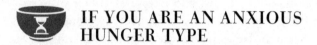

IF YOU ARE AN ANXIOUS HUNGER TYPE

You eat to distract yourself from anxiety and worry. You may snack compulsively or mindlessly; for example, while watching TV or when using a computer. The food you choose may not be high calorie. It could be very healthy, but the amount and frequency of eating has caused you to gain weight. A shortage of the hormone GABA or an excess of the hormone histamine or acetylcholine mean you may have physical symptoms such as allergies, headaches, a fast heartbeat or IBS. Eating large meals is your effort to calm yourself down, although this will exacerbate IBS.

What you need to do

❯ Boost your magnesium level, as this is a natural sedative. Eat more green vegetables.

❯ Choose foods that contain glutamic acid, as this helps you make the calming brain hormone GABA. Good sources are almonds, oats, halibut, mackerel and brown rice.

❯ Drink green tea, as this contains less caffeine and more of the amino acid L-theanine, which is known to have a tranquilizing effect.

❯ Balance your blood sugar to stabilize your mood. Replace simple carbohydrates, such as candy, chocolate, cakes, cookies, white rice, pasta and bread, with whole grains.

❯ Learn to meditate or consider hypnosis, counseling or cognitive behavioral therapy (CBT) to help you reduce your anxieties.

❯ Do the 48-Hour Hunger Rehab.

❯ Follow the 14-Day Anxious Hunger Weight Loss Food Plan, which starts on the next page.

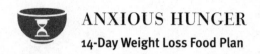

ANXIOUS HUNGER
14-Day Weight Loss Food Plan

	Day 1	Day 2	Day 3
Breakfast	Homemade Microwave Oatmeal (p. 200) with Green Banana and Walnut Topping (p. 205)	Bran and Berry Muffin (p. 193)	Homemade Microwave Oatmeal (p. 200) with Blueberry Protein Boost (p. 204)
Lunch	Chinese Pork and Spinach Broth (p. 237)	Eastern Chickpea, Coconut and Spinach Lunch Pot (p. 268)	Brown Rice Wrap (p. 256) with Tuna with a Kick (p. 259)
Snack (optional)	Vanilla Frozen Yogurt (p. 290) and sunflower seeds	Pepitas Calientes (p. 288)	Broiled Pear with Ricotta and Cinnamon (p. 284)
Main meal	Mushroom and Lentil Stew with Tofu (p. 326)	Mini Fish Pie with Oaty Crumble Topping (p. 331)	Puy Lentil Salad with Goat's Cheese and Rosewater Dressing (p. 306)

Day 4	Day 5	Day 6	Day 7
Pecan Pancakes with Crispy Bacon (p. 219)	Almond and Coconut Oatmeal with Raspberry Swirl (p. 208)	Quinoa, Almond and Pumpkin Seed Toast (p. 210) with Healthier Chocolate and Hazelnut Spread (p. 214)	Overnight Slow-Cooker Raisin Oatmeal (p. 201)
Spelt and Seed Loaf Sandwich (p. 252) with Cottage Cheese and Walnut Slaw (p. 263)	Provençale Tuna and Ratatouille Lunch Pot (p. 266)	Zucchini and White Bean Soup (p. 243)	Dhal with Broccoli Lunch Pot (p. 269)
Veg sticks with Higher-Protein Hummus (p. 275)	Tangy Sunflower Seeds (p. 286)	Pepitas Calientes (p. 288)	Veg sticks with Spinach and Parmesan Dip (p. 278)
Turkish Eggs with Tomato and Garlic Yogurt (p. 315)	Posh Sardines on Toast (p. 308)	Spaghetti with Chargrilled Squid and Caponata (p. 323)	Tamarind-Glazed Chicken Salad (p. 301)

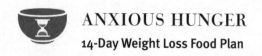

ANXIOUS HUNGER

14-Day Weight Loss Food Plan

	Day 8	Day 9	Day 10
Breakfast	Quinoa, Almond and Pumpkin Seed Toast (p. 210) with Avocado Butter (p. 212)	Strawberry and Oatmeal Smoothie (p. 190)	Homemade Microwave Oatmeal (p. 200) with Apple and Vanilla Sauce (p. 202)
Lunch	Mackerel Salad with Creamy Horseradish Dressing (p. 231)	Sweet-and-Sour Pork Lunch Pot (p. 265)	Edamame and Basil Soup (p. 244)
Snack (optional)	Veg sticks with Red Bell Pepper Dip (p. 274)	Spiced Almonds (p. 287)	Veg sticks with Spinach and Parmesan Dip (p. 278)
Main meal	Poached Egg with Edamame and Kale (p. 314)	Butter Bean, Parmesan and Thyme Burger (p. 312)	Feel-Good Chili (p. 320)

Day 11	Day 12	Day 13	Day 14
Oat and Almond Power Balls (p. 196)	Homemade Microwave Oatmeal (p. 200) with Spiced Pear and Prune Compote (p. 203)	Coconut Pancakes with Black Forest Drizzle (p. 220)	Homemade Microwave Oatmeal (p. 200) with Chocolate and Chili Melt (p. 206)
Spelt and Seed Loaf Sandwich (p. 252) with Thai-Style Crayfish and Cucumber (p. 261)	Tuscan Tomato Soup (p. 245)	Feta, Walnut and Pomegranate Salad (p. 234)	Spicy Lentil Soup (p. 247)
Broiled Pear with Ricotta and Cinnamon (p. 284)	Tangy Sunflower Seeds (p. 286)	Veg Sticks with Higher-Protein Hummus (p. 275)	Vanilla Frozen Yogurt (p. 290)
Tuna Steak with Fava Beans, Snow Peas and Oregano Oil (p. 322)	Red Mullet, Almond and Fennel Salad with Blood Orange Dressing (p. 304)	Tofu and Beet Burger (p. 313)	Roasted Vegetables with Broccoli and Pomegranate Couscous (p. 333)

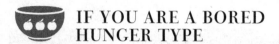 # IF YOU ARE A BORED HUNGER TYPE

Food is a displacement activity for you. Eating is something to do to fill downtime. You may not overeat at meals, largely since you aren't that hungry because you have snacked so much in between. The kind of food you eat will be whatever is there—in the fridge or cupboards. You are not driven by specific cravings. You can even overeat on really healthy foods, but too much of anything—even rice cakes—causes weight gain. You may also have Cravings (see page 33) and/ or Emotional Hunger (see page 41), or you may have just got into the habit of eating mindlessly.

What you need to do

> Remove high-calorie snack foods, such as cookies and potato chips, from your home, as these may be the first foods you reach for. If you have children, at least move these foods so that they are not at your eye level. Move tempting foods up or down in the fridge or to the back of cupboards.

> Make yourself some fresh and healthy snacks instead—raw veg sticks with low-fat dips or soup, for example, so that if you just have to graze you won't do too much damage.

> Have a "no standing up or lying down to eat" rule. Decide only to eat sitting down at a table with a knife and fork. No eating straight from the fridge or cupboards, on the sofa, in bed or in the car.

> Separate yourself from your food source by going out. Take up a hobby that gets you out of the home—hiking, swimming, gardening—or arrange to meet up with friends for a (non-food) treat.

> Do the 48-Hour Hunger Rehab.

> Follow the 14-Day Cravings Hunger Weight Loss Food Plan (starting on page 106) or the 14-Day Emotional Hunger Weight Loss Food Plan (starting on page 112) and refer back to Bored Hunger on page 31.

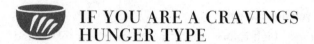

IF YOU ARE A CRAVINGS HUNGER TYPE

Your efforts to diet in the past may have been sabotaged by cravings for things like chocolate, cake, cookies, ice cream or other high-fat, high-sugar foods. Your cravings don't have to be sweet. Cheese Sandwiches and pizza also fall into this category, because starchy foods such as bread, pasta and rice also break down into fat in the body; however, it is more common for the foods you love to be types of desserts.

What you need to do

> Balance your blood sugar to strengthen you against "weak" moments when you are more likely to give in to cravings. Replace simple carbohydrates, such as candy, chocolate, cakes, cookies, white rice, pasta and bread, with whole grains.

> Choose foods that are a source of the amino acid L-tyrosine, as this helps you make dopamine, the brain hormone you may be low in. Eat very low-fat cottage cheese or ricotta cheese, yogurt, chicken, turkey, duck, venison, oats and dark chocolate.

> Avoid junk foods, such as candy and milk chocolate, cake, cookies and ice cream.

> Take a multivitamin containing iron, magnesium, copper, vitamin C and B complex to supply the micronutrients you need to make dopamine.

> Reduce your stress levels, eat regularly and get enough sleep. Try not to get hungry, angry, lonely or tired, as these states weaken you to cravings.

> Do the 48-Hour Hunger Rehab.

> Follow the 14-Day Cravings Hunger Weight Loss Food Plan, which starts on the next page.

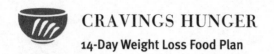

CRAVINGS HUNGER
14-Day Weight Loss Food Plan

	Day 1	Day 2	Day 3
Breakfast	Homemade Microwave Oatmeal (p. 200) with Green Banana and Walnut Topping (p. 205)	Mushroom Rarebit (p. 221)	Oat and Almond Power Balls (p. 196)
Lunch	Healthy Shrimp Laksa (p. 242)	Spanish Fish Soup (p. 241)	Asian Slaw with Shrimp (p. 232)
Snack (optional)	Tangy Sunflower Seeds (p. 286)	Chocolate Frozen Yogurt (p. 291)	Spiced Almonds (p. 287)
Main meal	Tamarind-Glazed Chicken Salad (p. 301)	Feel-Good Chili (p. 320)	Mediterranean Eggs (p. 316)

Day 4	Day 5	Day 6	Day 7
Keralan Omelet with Tomato and Green Chili (p. 216)	Peanut Butter and Blueberry Smoothie (p. 189)	Pecan Pancakes with Crispy Bacon (p. 219)	Strawberry and Oatmeal Smoothie (p. 190)
Edamame and Basil Soup (p. 244)	Chinese Pork and Spinach Broth (p. 237)	Turkey and Broccoli Salad with Gremolata (p. 229)	Feta, Walnut and Pomegranate Salad (p. 234)
Melon and Ham Roll-Ups (p. 283)	Fastest-Ever Berry Frozen Yogurt (p. 292)	Veg sticks with Red Bell Pepper Dip (p. 274)	Guacamole Egg (p. 281)
Cajun Spiced Trout (p. 321)	Vietnamese Shaking-Beef Salad (p. 302)	Poached Eggs and Asparagus on Toast (p. 309)	Persian Chicken Skewer with Herbed Cauliflower Plaf (p. 327)

CRAVINGS HUNGER

14-Day Weight Loss Food Plan

	Day 8	Day 9	Day 10
Breakfast	Peanut Breakfast Bar (p. 195)	Chinese or Thai Omelet (p. 215)	Chocolate and Cherry Smoothie (p. 191)
Lunch	Spelt and Seed Loaf Sandwich (p. 252) with Cottage Cheese and Walnut Slaw (p. 263)	Shrimp, Quinoa and Paprika Paella Lunch Pot (p.267)	Thai Chicken and Mushroom Broth (p. 236)
Snack (optional)	Veg sticks with Smoked Salmon and Dill Dip (p. 273)	Eggs Nicosia (p. 280)	Veg sticks and Higher-Protein Hummus (p. 275)
Main meal	Venison with Dukkah Rub and Quinoa Salad (p. 328)	Turkey and Feta Burger (p. 310)	Boeuf Bourguignon with Broccoli Mash (p. 329)

Day 11	Day 12	Day 13	Day 14
Gingerbread Muffin (p. 192)	Omelet-a-Go-Go (p. 215)	Quinoa, Almond and Pumpkin Seed Toast (p. 210) with Healthier Chocolate and Hazelnut Spread (p. 214)	Coconut Pancakes with Black Forest Drizzle (p. 220)
Hungarian Beef and Beet Soup (p. 240)	Whole-Wheat Pita Bread (p. 255) with Marrakesh Chicken Salad (p. 257)	Chicken and Green Mango Salad (p. 228)	Miso Soup with Butternut Squash and Tofu (p. 250)
Broiled Pear with Ricotta and Cinnamon (p. 284)	Apple and Blue Cheese Melt (p. 285)	Pepitas Calientes (p. 288)	Veg sticks with Mustardy Butter Bean Dip (p. 276)
Poached Egg with Edamame and Kale (p. 314)	Spiced Tuna Burger (p. 311)	Salt-Crusted Sea Bass with Avocado and Zucchini Salad (p. 330)	Mini Fish Pie with Oaty Crumble Topping (p. 331)

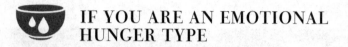

IF YOU ARE AN EMOTIONAL HUNGER TYPE

You are a classic "comfort eater", someone who eats when they are upset. You may also eat when you are angry, guilty, fearful or simply feeling down. You may have a family history of mild depression, or have been brought up to be a "coper", someone who soldiers on no matter what. Food is your emotional crutch, however. It helps you deal with difficult situations, people and emotions. This may be because you have sub-optimal levels of the natural antidepressant hormone serotonin in your body and so you crave starchy foods such as bread, potatoes and pasta, which lift serotonin.

What you need to do

❯ Eat healthy low-GI carbohydrate foods, such as brown rice, quinoa and oatmeal to supply the sugar to lift serotonin naturally and gently.

❯ Include foods that are a source of the amino acid tryptophan, which helps make the antidepressant and appetite-suppressant hormone serotonin in your daily diet. Turkey, chicken, reduced-fat cheese, milk and yogurt, eggs, fish and peanut butter are all good choices.

❯ Consider taking the herbal supplement 5-HTP, which helps you make serotonin. Take it at night on an empty stomach, at least two hours after supper, with a small glass of fruit juice to provide the sugar needed to potentiate its action.

❯ Exercise to boost your endorphins, which are also natural pain relievers but are calorie-free. Do 30 minutes of cardio, fast walking, running or cycling daily.

❯ Learn to "name" your emotions rather than pushing them down with food. When you feel bad, work out exactly which emotion you are feeling, and either write it down or say—or shout it—out loud: "I am ANGRY!"

❯ Do the 48-Hour Hunger Rehab.

❯ Follow the 14-Day Emotional Hunger Weight Loss Food Plan, which starts on the next page.

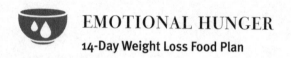

EMOTIONAL HUNGER
14-Day Weight Loss Food Plan

	Day 1	Day 2	Day 3
Breakfast	Homemade Microwave Oatmeal (p. 200) with Green Banana and Walnut Topping (p. 205)	Mexican Breakfast Tortilla (p. 217)	Chocolate and Cherry Smoothie (p. 191)
Lunch	Healthy Shrimp Laksa (p. 242)	Provençale Tuna and Ratatouille Lunch Pot (p. 266)	Mexican Pinto Bean Soup with Avocado Salsa (p. 248)
Snack (optional)	Pepitas Calientes (p. 288)	Apple and Blue Cheese Melt (p. 285)	Eggs Nicosia (p. 280)
Main meal	Feel-Good Chili (p. 320)	Tofu Mutter Paneer with Chapati (p. 324)	Persian Chicken Skewer with Herbed Cauliflower Plaf (p. 327)

Day 4	Day 5	Day 6	Day 7
Rye and Fennel Seed Toast (p. 211) with Reduced-Fat Peanut Butter (p. 213)	Overnight Slow-Cooker Raisin Oatmeal (p. 201)	Peanut Butter and Blueberry Smoothie (p. 189)	Surprise Chocolate Muffin (p. 194)
Chicken and Green Mango Salad (p. 228)	Ouillade (p. 238)	Cheat's Chicken Caesar Salad (p. 227)	Turkey and Broccoli Salad with Gremolata (p. 229)
Broiled Pear with Ricotta and Cinnamon (p. 284)	Veg sticks with Higher-Protein Hummus (p. 275)	All-Day Breakfast Egg (p. 279)	Veg sticks with Smoked Salmon and Dill Dip (p. 273)
Posh Sardines on Toast (p. 308)	Scallop and Green Papaya Salad (p. 305)	Tofu and Beet Burger (p. 313)	Poached Eggs and Asparagus on Toast (p. 309)

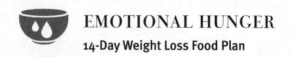

EMOTIONAL HUNGER
14-Day Weight Loss Food Plan

	Day 8	Day 9	Day 10
Breakfast	Homemade Microwave Oatmeal (p. 200) with Apple and Vanilla Sauce (p. 202)	Gingerbread Muffin (p. 192)	Quinoa, Almond and Pumpkin Seed Toast (p. 210) with Avocado Butter (p. 212)
Lunch	Moroccan Fava Bean Soup (p. 246)	Thai Chicken and Mushroom Broth (p. 236)	Sweet-and-Sour Pork Lunch Pot (p. 265)
Snack (optional)	Guacamole Egg (p. 281)	Veg sticks with Smoked Salmon and Dill Dip (p. 273)	Veg sticks with Higher-Protein Hummus (p. 275)
Main meal	Turkey and Feta Burger (p. 310)	Turkish Eggs with Tomato and Garlic Yogurt (p. 315)	Spaghetti with Chargrilled Squid and Caponata (p. 323)

Day 11	Day 12	Day 13	Day 14
Peanut Breakfast Bar (p. 195)	Strawberry and Oatmeal Smoothie (p. 190)	Homemade Microwave Oatmeal (p. 200) with Chocolate and Chili Melt (p. 206)	Oat and Almond Power Balls (p. 196)
Whole-Wheat Pita Bread (p. 255) with Marrakesh Chicken Salad (p. 257)	No-Knead Buckwheat Bread Sandwich (p. 253) with Turkey Cranberry (p. 258)	Tuscan Tomato Soup (p. 245)	Shrimp, Quinoa and Paprika Paella Lunch Pot (p. 267)
All-Day Breakfast Egg (p. 279)	Broiled Pear with Ricotta and Cinnamon (p. 284)	Eggs Nicosia (p. 280)	Apple and Blue Cheese Melt (p. 285)
Tuna Steak with Fava Beans, Snow Peas and Oregano Oil (p. 322)	Better BLT (p. 307)	Chicken Jalfrezi (p. 318)	Pork and Thyme Casserole (p. 319)

IF YOU ARE A HEDONISTIC HUNGER TYPE

Food is pleasure to you, which may be why you have always struggled with diets. You eat not because you are physically hungry, but because it tastes good, and if you really like something you can eat more and more of it. You have gotten into the habit of indulging yourself with fattening foods. These make you feel good, even if you hate the weight you have gained.

What you need to do:

> When eating meals, eat the food you like most first to prevent overeating.

> Slow down your eating. Put down your knife and fork between bites. This will allow the natural fullness signals from the hormone ghrelin to switch off your appetite.

> Include healthy fats and lean protein in every meal to increase satiety.

> Choose foods that are a source of the amino acid L-tyrosine, as this helps you make dopamine. Eat very low-fat cottage cheese or ricotta cheese, yogurt, chicken, turkey, duck, venison, oats and dark chocolate.

> Find other sources of pleasure. Spend time with friends and family, or take up a hobby you love.

> Do the 48-Hour Hunger Rehab.

> Follow the 14-Day Hedonistic Hunger Weight Loss Food Plan, which starts on the next page.

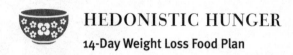

HEDONISTIC HUNGER

14-Day Weight Loss Food Plan

	Day 1	Day 2	Day 3
Breakfast	Rye and Fennel Seed Toast (p. 211) with Reduced-Fat Peanut Butter (p. 213)	Keralan Omelet with Tomato and Green Chili (p. 216)	Peanut Butter and Blueberry Smoothie (p. 189)
Lunch	Ouillade (p. 238)	Salmon and Avocado Salad with Wasabi Vinaigrette (p. 230)	Zucchini and White Bean Soup (p. 243)
Snack (optional)	Apple and Blue Cheese Melt (p. 285)	Fastest-Ever Berry Frozen Yogurt (p. 292)	Veg sticks with Spinach and Parmesan Dip (p. 278)
Main meal	Roasted Vegetables with Broccoli and Pomegranate Couscous (p. 333)	Butter Bean, Parmesan and Thyme Burger (p. 312)	Red Mullet, Almond and Fennel Salad with Blood Orange Dressing (p. 304)

Day 4	Day 5	Day 6	Day 7
Almond and Coconut Oatmeal with Raspberry Swirl (p. 208)	Coconut Pancakes with Black Forest Drizzle (p. 220)	Quinoa Crunch Bar (p. 197)	Overnight Slow-Cooker Raisin Oatmeal (p. 201)
Mexican Pinto Bean Soup with Avocado Salsa (p. 248)	Edamame and Basil Soup (p. 244)	Spicy Lentil Soup (p. 247)	Healthy Shrimp Laksa (p. 242)
Broiled Pear with Ricotta and Cinnamon (p. 284)	Veg sticks with Red Bell Pepper Dip (p. 274)	Veg sticks with Higher-Protein Hummus (p. 275)	Candied Lemons with Coconut (p. 293)
Turkish Eggs with Tomato and Garlic Yogurt (p. 315)	Tuna Steak with Fava Beans, Snow Peas and Oregano Oil (p. 322)	Turkey and Feta Burger (p. 310)	Puy Lentil Salad with Goat's Cheese and Rosewater Dressing (p. 306)

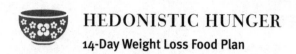

HEDONISTIC HUNGER
14-Day Weight Loss Food Plan

	Day 8	Day 9	Day 10
Breakfast	Strawberry and Oatmeal Smoothie (p. 190)	Quinoa, Almond and Pumpkin Seed Toast (p. 210) with Avocado Butter (p. 212)	Peanut Breakfast Bar (p. 195)
Lunch	Mackerel Salad with Creamy Horseradish Dressing (p. 231)	Provençale Tuna and Ratatouille Lunch Pot (p. 266)	Feta, Walnut and Pomegranate Salad (p. 234)
Snack (optional)	Veg sticks with Red Bell Pepper Dip (p. 274)	Apple and Blue Cheese Melt (p. 285)	Veg sticks with Higher-Protein Hummus (p. 275)
Main meal	Greek Vegetable and Halloumi Stew (p. 325)	Tofu and Beet Burger (p. 313)	Vietnamese Shaking-Beef Salad (p. 302)

Day 11	Day 12	Day 13	Day 14
Homemade Microwave Oatmeal (p. 200) with Apple and Vanilla Sauce (p. 202)	Pecan Pancakes with Crispy Bacon (p. 219)	Overnight Breakfast Roll with Scrambled Eggs and Smoked Salmon (p. 222)	Oat and Almond Power Balls (p. 196)
Brown Rice Wrap (p. 256) with Tuna with a Kick (p. 259)	Thai Chicken and Mushroom Broth (p. 236)	Miso Soup with Butternut Squash and Tofu (p. 250)	Asian Slaw with Shrimp (p. 232)
Broiled Pear with Ricotta and Cinnamon (p. 284)	Veg sticks with Spinach and Parmesan Dip (p. 278)	Candied Lemons with Coconut (p. 293)	Veg sticks with Smoked Salmon and Dill Dip (p. 273)
Mediterranean Eggs (p. 316)	Mushroom and Lentil Stew with Tofu (p. 326)	Cajun Spiced Trout (p. 321)	Butter Bean, Parmesan and Thyme Burger (p. 312)

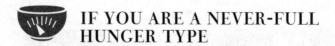

IF YOU ARE A NEVER-FULL HUNGER TYPE

Your hunger has a physical rather than an emotional cause. You can eat a meal, but you still don't feel full, so your portion sizes might be quite large in an effort to get that satisfied feeling. As a result, you may have gained quite a lot of weight. As a consequence of your weight gain, you may have been diagnosed with insulin resistance, high blood pressure or arthritis, so you have good reasons to reduce it, but diets are hard for you, as you feel constantly hungry. You fear not being full. The problem for you might be an imbalance in two key hormones: leptin and ghrelin.

What you need to do

> Eat a low-GI diet, which is one comprised of lean protein, good fats and slow-releasing carbs, as this has been shown to lift the level of the fullness hormone cholecystokinin.

> Eat high-volume, low-calorie foods, such as raw vegetables and salad. This will stretch the stomach, triggering the fullness hormone ghrelin.

> Eat chicory, which contains the fermentable fiber inulin, which may switch on the fullness hormone POMC.

> Make soup. Soup stays in the stomach for longer than solid food, so it will help you to feel satisfied.

> Pay attention to your hunger signals by completing the Hunger Scale (see page 174) before and during every meal. Switch off the TV and play some calming music to slow your eating down.

> Do the 48-Hour Hunger Rehab.

> Follow the 14-Day Never-Full Hunger Weight Loss Food Plan, which starts on the next page.

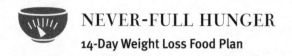

NEVER-FULL HUNGER
14-Day Weight Loss Food Plan

	Day 1	Day 2	Day 3
Breakfast	Almond and Coconut Oatmeal with Raspberry Swirl (p. 208)	Peanut Breakfast Bar (p. 195)	Homemade Microwave Oatmeal (p. 200) with Green Banana and Walnut Topping (p. 205)
Lunch	Ouillade (p. 238)	Eastern Chickpea, Coconut and Spinach Lunch Pot (p. 268)	Thai Chicken and Mushroom Broth (p. 236)
Snack (optional)	Pepitas Calientes (p. 288)	Spiced Almonds (p. 287)	Veg sticks with Higher-Protein Hummus (p. 275)
Main meal	Mushroom and Lentil Stew with Tofu (p. 326)	Mini Fish Pie with Oaty Crumble Topping (p. 331)	Scallop and Green Papaya Salad (p. 305)

Day 4	Day 5	Day 6	Day 7
Omelet-a-Go-Go (p. 215)	Quinoa Crunch Bar (p. 197)	Chocolate and Cherry Smoothie (p. 191)	Quinoa Oatmeal with Rhubarb and Ginger Jam (p. 209)
Whole-Wheat Pita Bread (p. 255) with Updated Shrimp Cocktail (p. 260)	Healthy Shrimp Laksa (p. 242)	Cheat's Chicken Caesar Salad (p. 227)	Tuscan Tomato Soup (p. 245)
Veg sticks with Mustardy Butter Bean Dip (p. 276)	Veg sticks with Red Bell Pepper Dip (p. 274)	Tangy Sunflower Seeds (p. 286)	Veg sticks with Spinach and Parmesan Dip (p. 278)
Feel-Good Chili (p. 320)	Butter Bean, Parmesan and Thyme Burger (p. 312)	Cod and Lychee Salad with Miso Dressing (p. 303)	Pork and Thyme Casserole (p. 319)

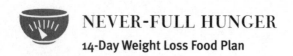

NEVER-FULL HUNGER

14-Day Weight Loss Food Plan

	Day 8	Day 9	Day 10
Breakfast	Mexican Breakfast Tortilla (p. 217)	Super-Seed Barley Oatmeal (p. 207)	Surprise Chocolate Muffin (p. 194)
Lunch	Shrimp, Quinoa and Paprika Paella Lunch Pot (p. 267)	Hungarian Beef and Beet Soup (p. 240)	Turkey and Broccoli Salad with Gremolata (p. 229)
Snack (optional)	Spiced Almonds (p. 287)	Tangy Sunflower Seeds (p. 286)	Veg sticks with Red Bell Pepper Dip (p. 274)
Main meal	Puy Lentil Salad with Goat's Cheese and Rosewater Dressing (p. 306)	Roasted Vegetables with Broccoli and Pomegranate Couscous (p. 333)	Greek Vegetable and Halloumi Stew (p. 325)

Day 11	Day 12	Day 13	Day 14
Homemade Microwave Oatmeal (p. 200) with Blueberry Protein Boost (p. 204)	Oat and Almond Power Balls (p. 196)	Strawberry and Oatmeal Smoothie (p. 190)	Coconut Pancakes with Black Forest Drizzle (p. 220)
Moroccan Fava Bean Soup (p. 246)	Asian Slaw with Shrimp (p. 232)	Dhal with Broccoli Lunch Pot (p. 269)	Mexican Pinto Bean Soup with Avocado Salsa (p. 248)
Veg sticks with Spinach and Parmesan Dip (p. 278)	Pepitas Calientes (p. 288)	Veg sticks with Warm Mexican Bean Dip (p. 277)	Vanilla Frozen Yogurt (p. 290)
Tuna Steak with Fava Beans, Snow Peas and Oregano Oil (p. 322)	Tofu and Beet Burger (p. 313)	Venison with Dukkah Rub and Quinoa Salad (p. 328)	Red Mullet, Almond and Fennel Salad with Blood Orange Dressing (p. 304)

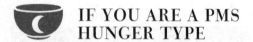

IF YOU ARE A PMS HUNGER TYPE

You may eat healthily most of the time, but things go downhill rapidly in the second half of your cycle. In the week before your period, your appetite increases and you crave chocolate and sugary snacks, such as cookies, as well as caffeine (tea/coffee/diet cola). As a result, your energy and mood may be unstable and you might feel tearful, angry or tired. You will also probably feel quite bloated, and this may make you feel even more down, leading you to eat even more. The problem is caused by the natural hormonal dip that happens before your period, but this could be being exacerbated by estrogen dominance.

What you need to do

> Balance your blood sugar to stabilize your hormones. Swap fast-releasing carbohydrates for whole grains. Include protein and some good fats in every meal and reduce stimulants such as tea/coffee/diet cola/alcohol.

> Increase your fiber intake by eating vegetables, beans and whole grains. Fiber helps with the excretion of "old" hormones such as estrogen, thus helping to balance circulating hormones better and avoid estrogen dominance.

> Support your liver. This is your body's principal organ of detoxification and helps with the excretion of "old" hormones. Include liver-friendly sulfurous vegetables such as broccoli, cauliflower and cabbage in your meals.

> Avoid headache tablets, indigestion tablets, food additives (such as MSG—monosodium glutamate), caffeine and alcohol. These all contribute to toxic load, which may over-tax the liver, making it less effective at processing the "old" estrogen.

> Take exercise. You may not feel like it in the week before your period, but cardio (fast walking, running, swimming and cycling) will stretch out tense muscles and increase endorphins, which have an antidepressant effect.

> Do the 48-Hour Hunger Rehab.

> Follow the 14-Day PMS Hunger Weight Loss Food Plan, which starts on the next page.

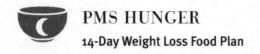

PMS HUNGER
14-Day Weight Loss Food Plan

	Day 1	Day 2	Day 3
Breakfast	Super-Seed Barley Oatmeal (p. 207)	Keralan Omelet with Tomato and Green Chili (p. 216)	Quinoa, Almond and Pumpkin Seed Toast (p. 210) with Avocado Butter (p. 212)
Lunch	Shrimp, Quinoa and Paprika Paella Lunch Pot (p. 267)	Zucchini and White Bean Soup (p. 243)	Dhal with Broccoli Lunch Pot (p. 269)
Snack (optional)	Eggs Nicosia (p. 280)	Spiced Almonds (p. 287)	Veg sticks with Smoked Salmon and Dill Dip (p. 273)
Main meal	Puy Lentil Salad with Goat's Cheese and Rosewater Dressing (p. 306)	Mini Fish Pie with Oaty Crumble Topping (p. 331)	Feel-Good Chili (p. 320)

Day 4	Day 5	Day 6	Day 7
Homemade Microwave Oatmeal (p. 200) with Blueberry Protein Boost (p. 204)	Omelet-a-Go-Go (p. 215)	Overnight Slow-Cooker Raisin Oatmeal (p. 201)	Quinoa Crunch Bar (p. 197)
Moroccan Fava Bean Soup (p. 246)	Turkey and Broccoli Salad with Gremolata (p. 229)	Salmon and Avocado Salad with Wasabi Vinaigrette (p. 230)	Asian Slaw with Shrimp (p. 232)
Tangy Sunflower Seeds (p. 286)	Veg sticks with Mustardy Butter Bean Dip (p. 276)	Veg sticks with Higher-Protein Hummus (p. 275)	Guacamole Egg (p. 281)
Cod and Lychee Salad with Miso Dressing (p. 303)	Japanese Marinated Tofu with Soba Noodles (p. 332)	Poached Egg with Edamame and Kale (p. 314)	Mushroom and Lentil Stew with Tofu (p. 326)

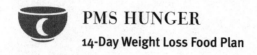

PMS HUNGER
14-Day Weight Loss Food Plan

	Day 8	Day 9	Day 10
Breakfast	Mushroom Rarebit (p. 221)	Quinoa Oatmeal with Rhubarb and Ginger Jam (p. 209)	Bran and Berry Muffin (p. 193)
Lunch	Mexican Pinto Bean Soup with Avocado Salsa (p. 248)	Spicy Lentil Soup (p. 247)	Spanish Fish Soup (p. 241)
Snack (optional)	Tangy Sunflower Seeds (p. 286)	Guacamole Egg (p. 281)	Veg sticks with Warm Mexican Bean Dip (p. 277)
Main meal	Spiced Tuna Burger (p. 311)	Better BLT (p. 307)	Roasted Vegetables with Broccoli and Pomegranate Couscous (p. 333)

Day 11	Day 12	Day 13	Day 14
Chinese or Thai Omelet (p. 215)	Rye and Fennel Seed Toast (p. 211) with Reduced-Fat Peanut Butter (p. 213)	Homemade Microwave Oatmeal (p. 200) with Chocolate and Chili Melt (p. 206)	Pecan Pancakes with Crispy Bacon (p. 219)
Ouillade (p. 238)	Mackerel Salad with Creamy Horseradish Dressing (p. 231)	Miso Soup with Butternut Squash and Tofu (p. 250)	Tuscan Tomato Soup (p. 245)
Pepitas Calientes (p. 288)	Spiced Almonds (p. 287)	Veg sticks with Higher-Protein Hummus (p. 275)	Veg sticks with Mustardy Butter Bean Dip (p. 276)
Scallop and Green Papaya Salad (p. 305)	Butter Bean, Parmesan and Thyme Burger (p. 312)	Persian Chicken Skewer with Herbed Cauliflower Plaf (p. 327)	Salt-Crusted Sea Bass with Avocado and Zucchini Salad (p. 330)

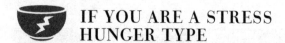 # IF YOU ARE A STRESS HUNGER TYPE

Your hunger is being driven by an increased stress response in your body. Either you have a highly stressful life (working long hours/multiple family responsibilities) or you have been through a period of extraordinary stress (separation/divorce/bereavement/illness). Your adrenals may be stressed, which means that you may feel tired all the time or only at certain times (on waking/at around 6 PM, for example), but you use food and stimulants (tea, coffee, diet cola, alcohol) to push yourself through these times.

What you need to do

> Nourish your adrenal glands with foods that are high in vitamin C, such as citrus fruits, guava, kiwi fruit, broccoli and bell peppers. Cook with parsley and thyme.

> Increase your intake of B vitamins to help your adrenals and to give you energy. Eat whole grains, beans and seeds.

> Include plenty of healthy fats to improve adrenal hormone function. Eat oily fish (salmon, trout, mackerel, sardines) and unsalted nuts and seeds, or dress your salad with flaxseed oil.

> Supplement with the herb rhodiola, which has been shown to block the stress response in the body.

> Reduce your stress, or learn to manage your stress better: eliminate, automate and delegate. Get rid of the "small stuff"; pay bills by direct debit and shop online; ask others to help you.

> Do the 48-Hour Hunger Rehab.

> Follow the 14-Day Stress Hunger Weight Loss Food Plan, which starts on the next page.

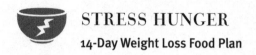

STRESS HUNGER
14-Day Weight Loss Food Plan

	Day 1	Day 2	Day 3
Breakfast	Rye and Fennel Seed Toast (p. 211) with Reduced-Fat Peanut Butter (p. 213)	Almond and Coconut Oatmeal with Raspberry Swirl (p. 208)	Peanut Butter and Blueberry Smoothie (p. 189)
Lunch	Dhal with Broccoli Lunch Pot (p. 269)	Provençale Tuna and Ratatouille Lunch Pot (p. 266)	Spelt and Seed Loaf Sandwich (p. 252) with Cottage Cheese and Walnut Slaw (p. 263)
Snack (optional)	Tangy Sunflower Seeds (p. 286)	Spiced Almonds (p. 287)	Veg sticks with Warm Mexican Bean Dip (p. 277)
Main meal	Spiced Tuna Burger (p. 311)	Tofu and Beet Burger (p. 313)	Venison with Dukkah Rub and Quinoa Salad (p. 328)

Day 4	Day 5	Day 6	Day 7
Super-Seed Barley Oatmeal (p. 207)	Homemade Microwave Oatmeal (p. 200) with Spiced Pear and Prune Compote (p. 203)	Gingerbread Muffin (p. 192)	Mexican Breakfast Tortilla (p. 217)
Whole-Wheat Pita Bread (p. 255) with Updated Shrimp Cocktail (p. 260)	Chinese Pork and Spinach Broth (p. 237)	Edamame and Basil Soup (p. 244)	Spelt and Seed Loaf Sandwich (p. 252) with Thai-Style Crayfish and Cucumber (p. 261)
Pepitas Calientes (p. 288)	Veg sticks with Mustardy Butter Bean Dip (p. 276)	Veg sticks with Red Bell Pepper Dip (p. 274)	Vanilla Frozen Yogurt (p. 290)
Butter Bean, Parmesan and Thyme Burger (p. 312)	Greek Vegetable and Halloumi Stew (p. 325)	Tofu Mutter Paneer with Chapati (p. 324)	Roasted Vegetables with Broccoli and Pomegranate Couscous (p. 333)

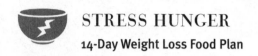

STRESS HUNGER
14-Day Weight Loss Food Plan

	Day 8	Day 9	Day 10
Breakfast	Quinoa Crunch Bar (p. 197)	Overnight Breakfast Roll with Scrambled Eggs and Smoked Salmon (p. 222)	Oat and Almond Power Balls (p. 196)
Lunch	Mexican Pinto Bean Soup with Avocado Salsa (p. 248)	Zucchini and White Bean Soup (p. 243)	Sweet-and-Sour Pork Lunch Pot (p. 265)
Snack (optional)	Pepitas Calientes (p. 288)	Veg sticks with Red Bell Pepper Dip (p. 274)	Vanilla Frozen Yogurt (p. 290)
Main meal	Pork and Thyme Casserole (p. 319)	Posh Sardines on Toast (p. 308)	Puy Lentil Salad with Goat's Cheese and Rosewater Dressing (p. 306)

Day 11	Day 12	Day 13	Day 14
Bran and Berry Muffin (p. 193)	Homemade Microwave Oatmeal (p. 200) with Green Banana and Walnut Topping (p. 205)	Quinoa, Almond and Pumpkin Seed Toast (p. 210) with Avocado Butter (p. 212)	Quinoa Oatmeal with Rhubarb and Ginger Jam (p. 209)
No-Knead Buckwheat Bread Sandwich (p. 253) with Spiced Egg Salad (p. 262)	Moroccan Fava Bean Soup (p. 246)	Turkey and Broccoli Salad with Gremolata (p. 229)	Spicy Lentil Soup (p. 247)
Veg sticks with Mustardy Butter Bean Dip (p. 276)	Candied Lemons with Coconut (p. 293)	Veg sticks with Warm Mexican Bean Dip (p. 277)	Tangy Sunflower Seeds (p. 286)
Spaghetti with Chargrilled Squid and Caponata (p. 323)	Red Mullet, Almond and Fennel Salad with Blood Orange Dressing (p. 304)	Mushroom and Lentil Stew with Tofu (p. 326)	Vietnamese Shaking-Beef Salad (p. 302)

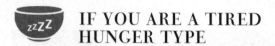

IF YOU ARE A TIRED HUNGER TYPE

Poor sleep is at the root of your weight gain. You may work shifts, travel or have a young baby who has you up at all hours, or perhaps you suffer from insomnia. Either way, this may have disrupted your circadian rhythm, which may mean you feel hungrier. Production of your natural sleep hormone melatonin and levels of serotonin may both be low, resulting in you feeling sleepy and a bit down, and further leading to overeating.

What you need to do

> Eat foods containing tryptophan, which will help you make both melatonin and serotonin. Choose turkey, chicken, low-fat cheese, eggs, milk, peanut butter, seeds, soya and tofu. Other key tryptophan foods include dates, papaya and banana.

> Cut your caffeine, especially after 12 noon, to improve sleep.

> Take a multivitamin–mineral supplement that includes magnesium, iron, calcium, zinc, vitamin C and vitamin B6 to support serotonin production.

> Get thicker curtains, and switch off lights, TV and computer screens in your bedroom to help melatonin production.

> Establish a sleep routine exactly as you would do for a baby. Try the three Bs—bath, bed, book. Go to bed and get up at the same time every day, including weekends.

> Do the 48-Hour Hunger Rehab.

> Follow the 14-Day Tired Hunger Weight Loss Food Plan, which starts on the next page.

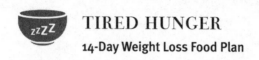

TIRED HUNGER

14-Day Weight Loss Food Plan

	Day 1	Day 2	Day 3
Breakfast	Quinoa, Almond and Pumpkin Seed Toast (p. 210) with Healthier Chocolate and Hazelnut Spread (p. 214)	Almond and Coconut Oatmeal with Raspberry Swirl (p. 208)	Bran and Berry Muffin (p. 193)
Lunch	Eastern Chickpea, Coconut and Spinach Lunch Pot (p. 268)	Whole-Wheat Pita Bread (p. 255) with Marrakesh Chicken Salad (p. 257)	Cheat's Chicken Caesar Salad (p. 227)
Snack (optional)	Tangy Sunflower Seeds (p. 286)	Guacamole Egg (p. 281)	Chocolate Frozen Yogurt (p. 291)
Main meal	Vietnamese Shaking-Beef Salad (p. 302)	Scallop and Green Papaya Salad (p. 305)	Tofu and Beet Burger (p. 313)

Day 4	Day 5	Day 6	Day 7
Homemade Microwave Oatmeal (p. 200) with Green Banana and Walnut Topping (p. 205)	Quinoa Crunch Bar (p. 197)	Homemade Microwave Oatmeal (p. 200) with Blueberry Protein Boost (p. 204)	Chocolate and Cherry Smoothie (p. 191)
Tuscan Tomato Soup (p. 245)	Hungarian Beef and Beet Soup (p. 240)	Chinese Pork and Spinach Broth (p. 237)	Sweet-and-Sour Pork Lunch Pot (p. 265)
Veg sticks with Smoked Salmon and Dill Dip (p. 273)	Pepitas Calientes (p. 288)	Eggs Nicosia (p. 280)	Veg sticks with Red Bell Pepper Dip (p. 274)
Turkey and Feta Burger (p. 310)	Turkish Eggs with Tomato and Garlic Yogurt (p. 315)	Red Mullet, Almond and Fennel Salad with Blood Orange Dressing (p. 304)	Posh Sardines on Toast (p. 308)

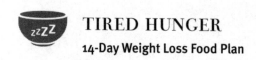

TIRED HUNGER
14-Day Weight Loss Food Plan

	Day 8	Day 9	Day 10
Breakfast	Peanut Butter and Blueberry Smoothie (p. 189)	Quinoa Oatmeal with Rhubarb and Ginger Jam (p. 209)	Quinoa, Almond and Pumpkin Seed Toast (p. 210) with Avocado Butter (p. 212)
Lunch	Chicken and Green Mango Salad (p. 228)	Turkey and Broccoli Salad with Gremolata (p. 229)	Feta, Walnut and Pomegranate Salad (p. 234)
Snack (optional)	Veg sticks with Spinach and Parmesan Dip (p. 278)	Veg sticks with Higher-Protein Hummus (p. 275)	Vanilla Frozen Yogurt (p. 290)
Main meal	Better BLT (p. 307)	Spaghetti with Chargrilled Squid and Caponata (p. 323)	Boeuf Bourguignon with Broccoli Mash (p. 329)

Day 11	Day 12	Day 13	Day 14
Homemade Microwave Oatmeal (p. 200) with Apple and Vanilla Sauce (p. 202)	Gingerbread Muffin (p. 192)	Strawberry and Oatmeal Smoothie (p. 190)	Surprise Chocolate Muffin (p. 194)
Thai Chicken and Mushroom Broth (p. 236)	Spelt and Seed Loaf Sandwich (p. 252) with Cottage Cheese and Walnut Slaw (p. 263)	Brown Rice Wrap (p. 256) with Tuna with a Kick (p. 259)	Whole-Wheat Pita Bread (p. 255) with Updated Shrimp Cocktail (p. 260)
Broiled Pear with Ricotta and Cinnamon (p. 284)	Melon and Ham Roll-Ups (p. 283)	Candied Lemons with Coconut (p. 293)	All-Day Breakfast Egg (p. 279)
Mushroom and Lentil Stew with Tofu (p. 326)	Cod and Lychee Salad with Miso Dressing (p. 303)	Tamarind-Glazed Chicken Salad (p. 301)	Persian Chicken Skewer with Herbed Cauliflower Plaf (p. 327)

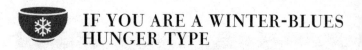

IF YOU ARE A WINTER-BLUES HUNGER TYPE

Your overeating is seasonal. It happens in the winter and is connected to the short, dark days. The lack of sunlight may be keeping your natural sleep hormone melatonin artificially high, which can make you feel groggy and unmotivated to do anything. Levels of the natural happy hormone serotonin may also be low, depressing your mood and leading you to crave sugar. Feelings of depression may be made worse by low levels of the sunshine vitamin, vitamin D.

What you need to do

> Boost serotonin levels nutritionally with food by eating tryptophan-rich foods like turkey, chicken, low-fat dairy and eggs. Instant tryptophan pick-me-ups include dates, papaya and banana.

> Eat foods that are both a source of essential fats to support brain function and which boost vitamin D, such as eggs and oily fish (like mackerel, sardines and salmon), cheese and mushrooms.

> Get outside, even in winter. Roll up your sleeves and let the available sunlight reach your skin to make vitamin D.

> Consider investing in an SAD lamp or an alarm clock that wakes you with light.

> Take the supplement 5-HTP in winter, as this can help to boost serotonin. Take it at night, on an empty stomach, at least two hours after dinner, with a small glass of fruit juice to boost its effect.

> Do the 48-Hour Hunger Rehab

> Follow the 14-Day Winter-Blues Hunger Weight Loss Food Plan, which starts on the next page.

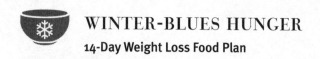

WINTER-BLUES HUNGER
14-Day Weight Loss Food Plan

	Day 1	Day 2	Day 3
Breakfast	Quinoa, Almond and Pumpkin Seed Toast (p. 210) with Avocado Butter (p. 212)	Peanut Breakfast Bar (p. 195)	Mushroom Rarebit (p. 221)
Lunch	Eastern Chickpea, Coconut and Spinach Lunch Pot (p. 268)	Whole-Wheat Pita Bread (p. 255) with Marrakesh Chicken Salad (p. 257)	Chicken and Green Mango Salad (p. 228)
Snack (optional)	Spiced Almonds (p. 287)	Apple and Blue Cheese Melt (p. 285)	Chocolate Frozen Yogurt (p. 291)
Main meal	Vietnamese Shaking-Beef Salad (p. 302)	Mini Fish Pie with Oaty Crumble Topping (p. 331)	Spiced Tuna Burger (p. 311)

Day 4	Day 5	Day 6	Day 7
Homemade Microwave Oatmeal (p. 200) with Chocolate and Chili Melt (p. 206)	Bran and Berry Muffin (p. 193)	Keralan Omelet with Tomato and Green Chili (p. 216)	Chocolate and Cherry Smoothie (p. 191)
Spanish Fish Soup (p. 241)	Provençale Tuna and Ratatouille Lunch Pot (p. 266)	Hungarian Beef and Beet Soup (p. 240)	Spelt and Seed Loaf Sandwich (p. 252) with Thai-Style Crayfish and Cucumber (p. 261)
Guacamole Egg (p. 281)	Broiled Pear with Ricotta and Cinnamon (p. 284)	Vanilla Frozen Yogurt (p. 290)	Veg sticks with Smoked Salmon and Dill Dip (p. 273)
Greek Vegetable and Halloumi Stew (p. 325)	Poached Eggs and Asparagus on Toast (p. 309)	Cod and Lychee Salad with Miso Dressing (p. 303)	Chicken Jalfrezi (p. 318)

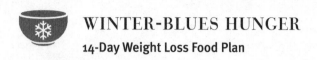

WINTER-BLUES HUNGER
14-Day Weight Loss Food Plan

	Day 8	Day 9	Day 10
Breakfast	Omelet-a-Go-Go (p. 215)	Gingerbread Muffin (p. 192)	Mexican Breakfast Tortilla (p. 217)
Lunch	Spelt and Seed Loaf Sandwich (p. 252) with Cottage Cheese and Walnut Slaw (p. 263)	Salmon and Avocado Salad with Wasabi Vinaigrette (p. 230)	Feta, Walnut and Pomegranate Salad (p. 234)
Snack (optional)	Vanilla Frozen Yogurt (p. 290)	Spiced Almonds (p. 287)	Veg sticks with Smoked Salmon and Dill Dip (p. 273)
Main meal	Cajun Spiced Trout (p. 321)	Mediterranean Eggs (p. 316)	Boeuf Bourguignon with Broccoli Mash (p. 329)

Day 11	Day 12	Day 13	Day 14
Peanut Butter and Blueberry Smoothie (p. 189)	Overnight Breakfast Roll with Scrambled Eggs and Smoked Salmon (p. 222)	Super-Seed Barley Oatmeal (p. 207)	Surprise Chocolate Muffin (p. 194)
No-Knead Buckwheat Bread Sandwich (p. 253) with Spiced Egg Salad (p. 262)	Edamame and Basil Soup (p. 244)	Mackerel Salad with Creamy Horseradish Dressing (p. 231)	Brown Rice Wrap (p. 256) with Tuna with a Kick (p. 259)
Chocolate Frozen Yogurt (p. 291)	Spiced Almonds (p. 287)	All-Day Breakfast Egg (p. 279)	Broiled Pear with Ricotta and Cinnamon (p. 284)
Posh Sardines on Toast (p. 308)	Venison with Dukkah Rub and Quinoa Salad (p. 328)	Tamarind-Glazed Chicken Salad (p. 301)	Tofu and Beet Burger (p. 313)

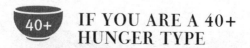

IF YOU ARE A 40+ HUNGER TYPE

You probably think it's harder to keep your weight down now than it used to be, and you would be right. Hormonal changes as a result of the perimenopause (women) and the andropause (men) may be causing both increased appetite and increased fat storage, especially around your middle. For women, the key hormones are estrogen and progesterone. For men, it's testosterone. Either way, you now gain weight and your mood may also be slightly depressed. A more sedentary lifestyle can also mean you are burning fewer calories.

What you need to do

> Boost your protein intake to balance your blood sugar and help conserve muscle mass to increase your metabolic rate. Older people process protein less effectively, so eat some low-fat dairy, eggs, meat or vegetable protein at every meal.

> Include healthy fats from oily fish (such as salmon, trout, mackerel and sardines) to improve the function of your sex hormones.

> Don't depress your thyroid. Over forties, particularly women, often have sub-optimal thyroid function, which can slow down their metabolism. Avoid soy milks and yogurt, tofu and soy sauce, as well as raw vegetables from the brassica family—that is, cabbage, kale, cauliflower and broccoli—as these can depress the thyroid.

> Take up weight training. This not only increases bone strength, which is important for older people, but it also builds muscle mass, which speeds up metabolism and fat burning.

> Do the 48-Hour Hunger Rehab.

> Follow the 14-Day 40+ Hunger Weight Loss Food Plan, which starts on the next page.

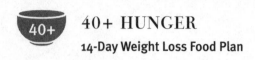

40+ HUNGER

14-Day Weight Loss Food Plan

	Day 1	Day 2	Day 3
Breakfast	Super-Seed Barley Oatmeal (p. 207)	Peanut Butter and Blueberry Smoothie (p. 189)	Mushroom Rarebit (p. 221)
Lunch	Salmon and Avocado Salad with Wasabi Vinaigrette (p. 230)	No-Knead Buckwheat Bread Sandwich (p. 253) with Spiced Egg Salad (p. 262)	Spanish Fish Soup (p. 241)
Snack (optional)	Broiled Pear with Ricotta and Cinnamon (p. 284)	Veg sticks with Higher-Protein Hummus (p. 275)	Fastest-Ever Berry Frozen Yogurt (p. 292)
Main meal	Poached Egg with Edamame and Kale (p. 314)	Spiced Tuna Burger (p. 311)	Roasted Vegetables with Broccoli and Pomegranate Couscous (p. 333)

Day 4	Day 5	Day 6	Day 7
Homemade Microwave Oatmeal (p. 200) with Blueberry Protein Boost (p. 204)	Chinese or Thai Omelet (p. 215)	Quinoa Crunch Bar (p. 197)	Coconut Pancakes with Black Forest Drizzle (p. 220)
Spicy Lentil Soup (p. 247)	Ouillade (p. 238)	Egg Salad with Spicy Tomato Dressing (p. 233)	Dhal with Broccoli Lunch Pot (p. 269)
Guacamole Egg (p. 281)	Veg sticks with Mustardy Butter Bean Dip (p. 276)	Veg sticks with Smoked Salmon and Dill Dip (p. 273)	Chocolate Frozen Yogurt (p. 291)
Posh Sardines on Toast (p. 308)	Japanese Marinated Tofu with Soba Noodles (p. 332)	Mediterranean Eggs (p. 316)	Cod and Lychee Salad with Miso Dressing (p. 303)

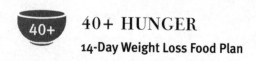

40+ HUNGER
14-Day Weight Loss Food Plan

	Day 8	Day 9	Day 10
Breakfast	Gingerbread Muffin (p. 192)	Omelet-a-Go-Go (p. 215)	Quinoa, Almond and Pumpkin Seed Toast (p. 210) with Avocado Butter (p. 212)
Lunch	Eastern Chickpea, Coconut and Spinach Lunch Pot (p. 268)	Shrimp, Quinoa and Paprika Paella Lunch Pot (p. 267)	Moroccan Fava Bean Soup (p. 246)
Snack (optional)	Eggs Nicosia (p. 280)	Veg sticks with Warm Mexican Bean Dip (p. 277)	Fastest-Ever Berry Frozen Yogurt (p. 292)
Main meal	Mini Fish Pie with Oaty Crumble Topping (p. 331)	Turkish Eggs with Tomato and Garlic Yogurt (p. 315)	Better BLT (p. 307)

Day 11	Day 12	Day 13	Day 14
Quinoa Oatmeal with Rhubarb and Ginger Jam (p. 209)	Strawberry and Oatmeal Smoothie (p. 190)	Overnight Breakfast Roll with Scrambled Eggs and Smoked Salmon (p. 222)	Pecan Pancakes with Crispy Bacon (p. 219)
Spelt and Seed Loaf Sandwich (p. 252) with Thai-Style Crayfish and Cucumber (p. 261)	Mackerel Salad with Creamy Horseradish Dressing (p. 231)	Miso Soup with Butternut Squash and Tofu (p. 250)	Edamame and Basil Soup (p. 244)
All-Day Breakfast Egg (p. 279)	Veg sticks with Mustardy Butter Bean Dip (p. 276)	Broiled Pear with Ricotta and Cinnamon (p. 284)	Veg sticks with Higher-Protein Hummus (p. 275)
Greek Vegetable and Halloumi Stew (p. 325)	Poached Eggs and Asparagus on Toast (p. 309)	Puy Lentil Salad with Goat's Cheese and Rosewater Dressing (p. 306)	Persian Chicken Skewer with Herbed Cauliflower Plaf (p. 327)

AT-A-GLANCE HUNGER TYPE RECIPES

Breakfast recipes	Anxious	Cravi
Peanut Butter and Blueberry Smoothie (p. 189)		*
Strawberry and Oatmeal Smoothie (p. 190)	*	*
Chocolate and Cherry Smoothie (p. 191)		*
Gingerbread Muffins (p. 192)		*
Bran and Berry Muffins (p. 193)	*	
Surprise Chocolate Muffins (p. 194)		
Peanut Breakfast Bars (p. 195)		*
Oat and Almond Power Balls (p. 196)	*	*
Quinoa Crunch Bars (p. 197)		*
Homemade Microwave Oatmeal (p. 200)	*	*
Overnight Slow-Cooker Raisin Oatmeal (p. 201)	*	
Apple and Vanilla Sauce (p. 202)	*	
Spiced Pear and Prune Compote (p. 203)	*	
Blueberry Protein Boost (p. 204)	*	
Green Banana and Walnut Topping (p. 205)	*	*
Chocolate and Chili Melt (p. 206)	*	
Super-Seed Barley Oatmeal (p. 207)		
Almond and Coconut Oatmeal with Raspberry Swirl (p. 208)	*	
Quinoa Oatmeal with Rhubarb and Ginger Jam (p. 209)		
Quinoa, Almond and Pumpkin Seed Bread (p. 210)	*	*
Rye and Fennel Seed Bread (p. 211)		
Avocado Butter (p. 212)	*	
Reduced-Fat Peanut Butter (p. 213)		*
Healthier Chocolate and Hazelnut Spread (p. 214)	*	*
Omelets-a-Go-Go (p. 215)		*
Chinese or Thai Omelet (p. 215)		*
Keralan Omelet with Tomato and Green Chili (p. 216)		*
Mexican Breakfast Tortilla (p. 217)		
Pecan Pancakes with Crispy Bacon (p. 219)	*	*
Coconut Pancakes with Black Forest Drizzle (p. 220)	*	*
Mushroom Rarebit (p. 221)		*
Overnight Breakfast Rolls with Scrambled Eggs and Smoked Salmon (p. 222)		

motional	Hedonistic	Never-Full	PMS	Stress	Tired	Winter-Blues	40+
★	★			★	★	★	★
★	★	★			★		★
★		★		★	★	★	
★			★	★	★	★	★
		★	★	★	★	★	
★		★			★	★	
★	★	★				★	★
★	★	★		★			
	★	★	★	★	★		★
★	★	★	★	★	★	★	★
★	★		★				
★	★				★		
		★		★			★
		★	★		★		★
★		★		★	★		
★			★			★	
		★	★	★		★	★
	★	★		★	★		
		★	★	★	★		★
★	★		★	★	★	★	★
★	★		★	★			
★	★		★	★	★	★	★
★	★		★	★	★	★	★
					★		
	★	★	★			★	★
	★	★	★			★	★
	★		★			★	
★		★		★		★	
	★		★	★			★
	★	★					★
			★			★	★
	★			★		★	★

Lunch recipes	Anxious	Cravin
Cheat's Chicken Caesar Salad (p. 227)		
Chicken and Green Mango Salad (p. 228)		*
Turkey and Broccoli Salad with Gremolata (p. 229)		*
Salmon and Avocado Salad with Wasabi Vinaigrette (p. 230)		
Mackerel Salad with Creamy Horseradish Dressing (p. 231)	*	
Asian Slaw with Shrimp (p. 232)		*
Egg Salad with Spicy Tomato Dressing (p. 233)		
Feta, Walnut and Pomegranate Salad (p. 234)	*	*
Thai Chicken and Mushroom Broth (p. 236)		*
Chinese Pork and Spinach Broth (p. 237)	*	*
Ouillade (p. 238)		
Hungarian Beef and Beet Soup (p. 240)		*
Spanish Fish Soup (p. 241)		*
Healthy Shrimp Laksa (p. 242)		*
Zucchini and White Bean Soup (p. 243)	*	
Edamame and Basil Soup (p. 244)	*	*
Tuscan Tomato Soup (p. 245)	*	
Moroccan Fava Bean Soup (p. 246)		
Spicy Lentil Soup (p. 247)	*	
Mexican Pinto Bean Soup with Avocado Salsa (p. 248)		
Miso Soup with Butternut Squash and Tofu (p. 250)		*
Spelt and Seed Loaf (p. 252)	*	*
No-Knead Buckwheat Bread (p. 253)		
Chickpea and Rosemary Bread (p. 254)	*	
Whole-Wheat Pita Bread (p. 255)		*
Brown Rice Wrap (p. 256)	*	
Marrakesh Chicken Salad (p. 257)		*
Turkey Cranberry (p. 258)		*
Tuna with a Kick (p. 259)	*	
Updated Shrimp Cocktail (p. 260)		
Thai-Style Crayfish and Cucumber (p. 261)	*	
Spiced Egg Salad (p. 262)		
Cottage Cheese and Walnut Slaw (p. 263)	*	*
Sweet-and-Sour Pork Lunch Pot (p. 265)	*	
Provençale Tuna and Ratatouille Lunch Pot (p. 266)	*	
Shrimp, Quinoa and Paprika Paella Lunch Pot (p. 267)		*
Eastern Chickpea, Coconut and Spinach Lunch Pot (p. 268)	*	
Dhal with Broccoli Lunch Pot (p. 269)	*	

Emotional	Hedonistic	Never-Full	PMS	Stress	Tired	Winter-Blues	40+
*		*			*		
*					*	*	
*		*	*	*	*		
	*		*			*	*
	*		*			*	*
	*	*	*				
*		*				*	*
	*				*		
*	*	*			*		
				*	*		
*	*	*	*				*
		*			*	*	
			*			*	*
*	*	*					
	*		*	*			
	*			*		*	*
*		*	*	*	*		
*		*	*		*		*
	*		*	*			*
*	*	*	*	*			
	*		*				*
				*	*	*	*
*			*	*	*	*	*
			*			*	*
*		*		*	*	*	
	*				*	*	
*					*	*	
*		*			*	*	*
	*				*	*	
	*	*		*	*		
			*	*		*	*
*			*	*	*	*	*
				*	*	*	
*				*	*		*
*	*	*		*		*	
*		*	*				*
		*			*	*	*
		*	*	*		*	*

Snack recipes	Anxious	Cravi
Smoked Salmon and Dill Dip (p. 273) (with veg sticks)		*
Red Bell Pepper Dip (p. 274) (with veg sticks)	*	*
Higher-Protein Hummus (p. 275) (with veg sticks)	*	*
Mustardy Butter Bean Dip (p. 276) (with veg sticks)	*	*
Warm Mexican Bean Dip (p. 277) (with veg sticks)		
Spinach and Parmesan Dip (p. 278) (with veg sticks)	*	
All-Day Breakfast Eggs (p. 279)		*
Eggs Nicosia (p. 280)		*
Guacamole Eggs (p. 281)		*
Melon and Ham Roll-Ups (p. 283)		*
Broiled Pear with Ricotta and Cinnamon (p. 284)	*	*
Apple and Blue Cheese Melt (p. 285)		*
Tangy Sunflower Seeds (p. 286)	*	*
Spiced Almonds (p. 287)	*	*
Pepitas Calientes (p. 288)	*	*
Vanilla Frozen Yogurt (p. 290)	*	*
Chocolate Frozen Yogurt (p. 291)		*
Fastest-Ever Berry Frozen Yogurt (p.292)		*
Candied Lemons with Coconut (p. 293)		
Chocolate and Hazelnut Thins with Sea Salt (p. 294)		*

Emotional	Hedonistic	Never-Full	PMS	Stress	Tired	Winter-Blues	40+
*	*		*		*	*	*
	*	*		*	*		
*	*	*	*		*		*
	*	*	*	*			*
		*	*	*			*
	*	*			*		
*					*	*	*
*			*		*		*
*			*		*	*	*
*					*		
*	*				*	*	*
*	*				*	*	*
		*	*	*	*		
		*	*	*		*	
*		*	*	*	*		*
		*		*	*	*	
		*			*	*	*
	*					*	*
	*		*	*	*		*
*		*	*		*	*	*

Main meal recipes	Anxious	Cravi
Tamarind-Glazed Chicken Salad (p. 301)	★	★
Vietnamese Shaking-Beef Salad (p. 302)		★
Cod and Lychee Salad with Miso Dressing (p. 303)		
Red Mullet, Almond and Fennel Salad with Blood Orange Dressing (p. 304)	★	
Scallop and Green Papaya Salad (p. 305)		
Puy Lentil Salad with Goat Cheese and Rosewater Dressing (p. 306)	★	
Better BLT (p. 307)		
Posh Sardines on Toast (p. 308)	★	
Poached Eggs and Asparagus on Toast (p. 309)		★
Turkey and Feta Burgers (p. 310)		★
Spiced Tuna Burgers (p. 311)		★
Butter Bean, Parmesan and Thyme Burgers (p. 312)	★	
Tofu and Beet Burgers (p. 313)	★	
Poached Eggs with Edamame and Kale (p. 314)	★	★
Turkish Eggs with Tomato and Garlic Yogurt (p. 315)	★	
Mediterranean Eggs (p. 316)	★	★
Chicken Jalfrezi (p. 318)		
Pork and Thyme Casserole (p. 319)		
Feel-Good Chilli (p. 320)	★	★
Cajun Spiced Trout (p. 321)		★
Tuna Steak with Fava Beans, Snow Peas and Oregano Oil (p. 322)	★	
Spaghetti with Chargrilled Squid and Caponata (p. 323)	★	
Tofu Mutter Paneer with Chapatis (p. 324)		
Greek Vegetable and Halloumi Stew (p. 325)		
Mushroom and Lentil Stew with Tofu (p. 326)	★	
Persian Chicken Skewers with Herbed Cauliflower Pilaf (p. 327)		★
Venison with Dukkah Rub and Quinoa Salad (p. 328)		★
Boeuf Bourguignon with Broccoli Mash (p. 329)		★
Salt-Crusted Sea Bass with Avocado and Zucchini Salad (p. 330)		★
Mini Fish Pie with Oaty Crumble Topping (p. 331)	★	★
Japanese Marinated Tofu with Soba Noodles (p. 332)		
Roasted Vegetables with Broccoli and Pomegranate Couscous (p. 333)	★	

Emotional	Hedonistic	Never-Full	PMS	Stress	Tired	Winter-Blues	40+
					*	*	
	*			*	*	*	
		*	*		*	*	*
	*	*		*	*		
*		*	*		*		
	*	*	*	*			*
*			*		*	*	*
*				*	*	*	*
*						*	*
*	*		*		*		
			*	*		*	*
	*	*	*	*			*
*	*	*		*	*	*	
			*				*
*	*				*		*
	*			*		*	*
*					*	*	
*		*		*			
*		*	*	*			
	*					*	*
*	*	*	*				*
*	*			*	*		
*				*	*		*
	*	*		*	*	*	*
	*	*	*	*	*		
*			*		*		*
		*		*		*	
					*	*	
*			*				
		*	*			*	*
*			*			*	*
	*	*	*	*	*		*

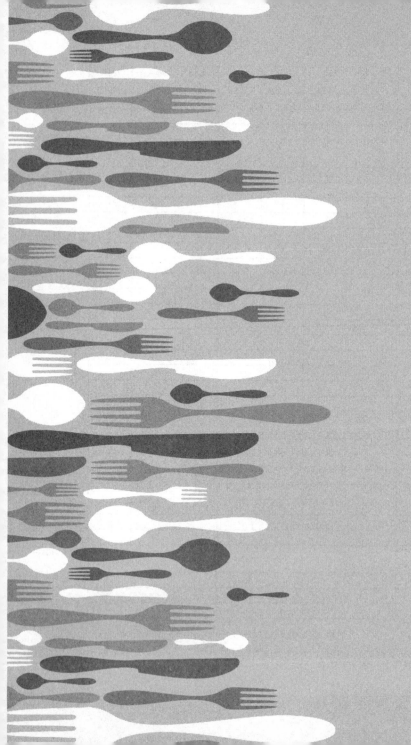

The 48-hour hunger rehab

One of the problems with there being so many different Hunger Types is that they can get all mixed up until you can barely tell whether you are really hungry at all. Either you feel hungry all the time, or you're never really hungry, but eat anyway.

Big swings in blood sugar due to feeding cravings or trying to use food to solve emotional issues can further lead to chaotic hunger signals. Reactive hypoglycemia, where you eat something high in sugar and then your blood sugar plunges down low again, can leave some people feeling jittery, and even sick, when they are hungry. In this state you do not make wise food choices. Your brain screams, "Chocolate brownie, NOW!", and you answer the call.

The Hunger Rehab is a 48-hour detox designed to help put you back in touch with your natural hunger signals. Instead of your normal routine of foods, you will be drinking healthy juices. I know, I know—this strikes terror into the heart of many. Don't worry, I'm not going to suggest body brushing, coffee enemas or eight hours silent meditation as well.

The point of the detox is not to torture you but to cleanse your body and clear your mind so that you can start your Hunger Type Food Plan free of some of the cravings and compulsions that may have been driving your eating.

The Hunger Rehab is useful because it:

> Gets you back in touch with your body's natural appetite and fullness signals
> Provides a break from the unhealthy food patterns that may have been causing your weight gain
> Reveals how much and what you were eating before so that you can identify the things you need to change
> Reduces unconscious eating by asking you to fill out a Hunger Scale
> Prevents compulsive eating by removing "addictive" foods, such as those that are high in fat and sugar
> Simplifies your life by reducing your food choices
> Removes sugar as a sedative, so it "wakes you up" to the emotional and psychological factors that may have been driving your eating
> Allows you to track your food–mood connection by getting you to complete a Mood and Food Diary
> Rebalances your system by balancing blood sugar and removing stimulants, such as tea, coffee and diet cola
> Nourishes your body so that all the systems can work more effectively
> Reduces bloating
> Kick-starts your weight loss

HOW MUCH WEIGHT WILL I LOSE ON THE HUNGER REHAB?

The primary aim of the Hunger Rehab is not weight loss but rebalancing. Your 14-Day Hunger Type Weight Loss Food Plan is the main weight-loss tool in this program; however, many people can lose significant amounts of weight on the Rehab, up to 5 pounds over 48 hours.

Some of this weight loss might be water. The reason is twofold. First, if you eat a lot of prepared foods or cook yourself adding salt, this can lead to water retention. There is no added salt (sodium) in the Hunger Rehab juices. Indeed, many are high in potassium, which buffers sodium in the body, offsetting its action and leading to water loss. By increasing potassium and reducing sodium, your body should naturally let go of excess water. You will look and feel slimmer quickly.

Second, if you have hidden food intolerances (often to wheat or dairy), your body may also retain water. The body dilutes what it regards as toxic, so you become bloated. The Hunger Rehab is wheat- and dairy-free, so you should lose water that way too.

WHAT IF I GET HUNGRY?

Well, that is the point, isn't it? I want you to feel hungry—not starving, but hungry—so that you can reconnect with what is a perfectly natural process. Hunger not only signals that you need to eat, but it also triggers the release of important hormones that manage body fat. If you never feel hungry, you will not lose weight. I want to stress here that I am not talking about extreme hunger. I do not want to promote eating disorders. The Hunger Rehab is designed for just 48 hours, not for life.

Extreme hunger can cause the release of endorphins, which is one reason why those with anorexia can actually feel good while starving themselves. But anorexia is life-threatening. Bulimia also has serious health risks, as does binge-eating disorder. If you think you have an eating disorder, please see a doctor.

The point about the Hunger Rehab is to reconnect you with your hunger signals and show you that these are not scary but manageable. If you are someone who has overeaten for a long time, it will also show you how much more pleasure you can get from eating when you are physically hungry.

Many overeaters fear hunger. I have had clients say to me anxiously, "Are you sure I'll feel full?", as if I am suggesting taking away a pacifier from a toddler. Food is their comfort blanket. They are all or nothing, thinking that if they actually feel hungry, it will be so overwhelming that they won't be able to cope. You can tell if you fall into this group if you always carry snacks with you wherever you go. Perhaps you plan journeys including when and where you will eat, or you make sure that your fridge and cupboards are always full. This behavior is redolent of panic, panic that the food will run out. But these days, unless you live in Timbuktu, there is always somewhere to buy food.

If the idea of hunger frightens you, it may be that what you fear is not overwhelming hunger but overwhelming emotion—sadness, anger, guilt and so on. The food is used to suppress these emotions in yourself, because if you were to start expressing them, you might not be able to stop. Alternatively, it may be that you have learned to fear emotion in others. Perhaps you had a parent who was prone to rages or depression?

In my experience with weight-loss clients, those who fear a shortage of food often grew up with a shortage of other things—time, love, attention or money. They had parents who, perhaps through no fault of their own, were busy, or absent physically or emotionally, or there were a lot of siblings.

I quite often see clients who have become overweight after a trauma—frequently some form of childhood abuse. One woman I remember told me that her parents cooked themselves meals and gave the children only the leftovers. At first, I didn't understand, but she explained that if her mother made a salad, she gave the children the cucumber peelings or the ends of the lettuce. They were never cooked a complete meal. No wonder my client and her brothers had gone on to binge as adults.

Still, I don't want to suggest that you have to have endured an *Angela's Ashes*-style appalling childhood to not want to be hungry. It is natural to desire being properly fed. Neither is carrying a bit of extra weight the sign of a damaged psyche. As I hope I have explained, there are all kinds of physical reasons why your body may not be working properly, and you may be either craving specific foods or storing more of what you eat as fat and gaining weight.

You don't have to do the Hunger Rehab if you really can't face it. The Hunger Type Weight Loss Food Plan will still work. And remember, if you do decide to do it, it's only 48 hours.

THE HUNGER SCALE

During the Hunger Rehab, it is important that you pay attention to your body; check and monitor how you are feeling. This is so that you can learn to recognize physical hunger and separate it from the other kinds of hunger that may have been driving your eating.

This may sound a bit daunting. If you're used to eating for a whole wealth of reasons, isolating the real hunger pangs and then deciding how "serious" they are is quite tricky. One very useful tool for doing this is the Hunger Scale. You should use it throughout the Hunger Rehab and indeed it may be a useful tool during your 14-Day Food Plan and beyond too.

The Hunger Scale

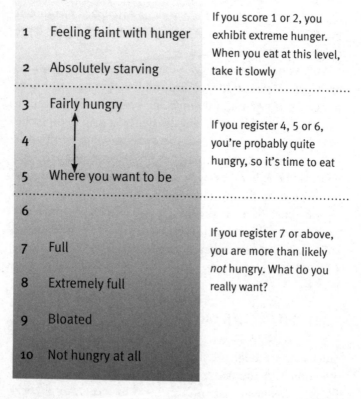

1	Feeling faint with hunger	If you score 1 or 2, you exhibit extreme hunger. When you eat at this level, take it slowly
2	Absolutely starving	
3	Fairly hungry	
4	↕	If you register 4, 5 or 6, you're probably quite hungry, so it's time to eat
5	Where you want to be	
6		
7	Full	If you register 7 or above, you are more than likely *not* hungry. What do you really want?
8	Extremely full	
9	Bloated	
10	Not hungry at all	

What you do is this: if you think you feel hungry, you get out your Hunger Scale and rate your hunger against it. Ideally, you want to be at about 3 or 4 to start eating. If you let yourself go as far as a 1 or 2, it is likely that you will overeat.

The Hunger Scale is equally helpful in telling you when to stop eating. As you eat, you do so slowly and continue to monitor your body. If you score 6 or 7 on the scale, you stop eating. If you still want to eat more, it's time to get out the Mood and Food Diary (more about that in a moment).

Of course, on the Hunger Rehab you are not eating, as such, you are drinking. As it is a low-calorie regime, you are likely to be more hungry than you normally would be. This should make those messages that might have become buried under piles of food in the past pretty easy to notice.

Persevere with the scale, as once you are on your 14-Day Hunger Type Weight Loss Food Plan, you should have gotten the hang of it, and it will be even more useful. When you go back to having a wider variety of things to "eat", you will need to remember to pay attention to your natural hunger and fullness signals to prevent overeating.

THE MOOD AND FOOD DIARY

This is another essential part of the Hunger Rehab. Remember: one of the reasons for doing it is to uncover emotions that may be driving your eating, and the Mood and Food Diary helps you with this. Of course, you will already have completed the What Hunger Type Are You? Quiz, so you may already know if you are an emotional eater; however, it's amazing how a detox can uncover buried emotions. Stripped of your usual food crutches (and we all have them), things come bubbling up.

I'm not trying to give you a mental breakdown here, but, if you do feel more emotional and even a bit teary during the Hunger Rehab, that is no bad thing. It may show you how you are much more reliant on eating as a coping strategy than for hunger. Filling in the diary also encourages you to think deeply about your feelings, which may be painful, but perhaps necessary. If the root of your hunger is a physical imbalance—estrogen dominance, adrenal stress, underactive thyroid, for example—the Mood and Food Diary has an added function. It will help to record how you could feel without your usual self-medication.

If you are under a lot of stress, for example, and you have been using sugar and caffeine to get yourself through the day, completing the Mood and Food Diary during the 48 hours you are juicing will reveal the true state of your health. Either it will show you how absolutely exhausted you are, or it will reveal how much better you can feel if you avoid the energy-and-mood sugar roller coaster. Either way, it provides motivation to change your eating.

The Mood and Food Diary has one last important job—to identify eating triggers. Because you have to record how you are feeling, it shows which people, places or things may make you want to eat.

Keep your diary with you all the time, as it's really important to record how you are feeling at the time, not trying to remember how you felt in the past.

Here's an idea of how to fill in your Mood and Food Diary.

Date and time	Saturday 8 AM	Sunday 9 PM
Where am I and what am I doing?	In bed	On the sofa, watching TV
Who am I with?	My partner	On my own
What emotion am I feeling?	Tired	Bored and dreading work tomorrow
What would I normally eat/drink now?	Go out for brunch —large latte and almond croissant	Packet of Doritos and dip, if being bad, or hummus and rice cakes, if being good
What do I actually eat/drink?	Juice	Juice
How do I feel afterwards?	Still tired, angry that I can't have my "treat"	Proud of myself for sticking to the diet. Glad the detox is almost over

OK, now you're ready for your Hunger Rehab.

HUNGER REHAB—THE RULES

1   Drink six juices per day. Drink only the juices and have no other food.

2   Go for variety. You can choose which juices to have, but do not have the same one over and over. Try a different one at every "meal" to ensure you get a range of nutrients.

3   Have your juices every three hours. Don't be tempted to save up your calories.

4   Drink plenty of water (eight glasses per day is recommended) or drink herbal/green tea. Avoid "normal" tea, coffee, carbonated drinks and all alcohol.

5   Exercise for at least 30 minutes per day, preferably outside. Walk, run, cycle or swim, for example.

6   Get plenty of sleep, seven to eight hours per night.

7   Do the Hunger Scale before and during eating. Complete your Mood and Food Diary at least four times per day.

8   Don't cheat.

THE HUNGER REHAB RECIPES

To make some of these recipes you will need a juicer. This will enable you to juice vegetables, which will keep your blood sugar more stable than fruit juices alone; however, I know that not everyone has a juicer, and they're pretty pricey to buy, so I have included other juices that can be made in a blender or food processor. If you have a juicer, you can select from both lists; if not, just stick with the blender/food processor recipes. Remember to vary your choice throughout the 48 hours to ensure a variety of nutrients.

Juicer recipes

Hunger Rehab Juice 1—Apple, Carrot and Ginger

Serves 1

3 apples
2 carrots
½ inch piece of ginger root, peeled

Put all the ingredients through an electric juicer, then serve the juice immediately.

Hunger Rehab Juice 2—Super-Greens

Serves 1

¼ pineapple
1 small bunch of watercress
2 broccoli florets
1 small bunch parsley
1 celery stalk

Cut off the skin from the pineapple, making sure you remove all the "eyes". Put all the ingredients through an electric juicer, then serve the juice immediately.

Hunger Rehab Juice 3—Beet and Orange

Serves 1

½ raw beet
juice of 3 oranges
a squeeze of lemon juice

Put the beet through an electric juicer, then stir in the orange and lemon juice. Serve the juice immediately.

Hunger Rehab Juice 4—Tomato and Celery

Serves 1

3 tomatoes
1 celery stalk
½ red bell pepper

Put all the ingredients through an electric juicer, then serve the juice immediately.

Hunger Rehab Juice 5—Coconut Water and Kale

Serves 1

1 small handful kale leaves
generous ⅓ cup pineapple juice
½ cup coconut water
¼ avocado, cut in half, pitted and
    peeled
a squeeze of lemon juice

Put the kale through an electric juicer, then transfer to a blender or food processor and add the other ingredients. Blend until smooth, then serve the juice immediately.

Blender/food processor recipes

Hunger Rehab Juice 6—Avocado and Mango

Serves 1

juice of 2 oranges
¼ avocado, cut in half, pitted and peeled
¼ mango, peeled, pitted and cut into chunks

Put all the ingredients into a blender or food processor and blend until smooth and creamy. Serve the juice immediately.

Hunger Rehab Juice 7—Melon and Cucumber

Serves 1

¼ honeydew melon, seeded
½ cucumber, peeled

Cut the melon flesh away from the peel. Discard the peel and cut the flesh into chunks. Cut the cucumber in half and scrape out the seeds. Put all the ingredients into a blender or food processor and blend until smooth. Serve the juice immediately.

Hunger Rehab Juice 8—Papaya and Lime

Serves 1

½ papaya, peeled, seeded and cut into chunks
juice of ½ lime
1 cup chilled coconut water

Put all the ingredients into a blender or food processor and blend until smooth. Serve the juice immediately.

Hunger Rehab Juice 9—Pear and Ginger

Serves 1

3 pears, peeled, cored and cut into chunks
¼ inch piece of ginger root, peeled and grated

Put the ingredients into a blender or food processor and blend until smooth. Serve immediately.

DAILY SCHEDULE

Drink your juices at the following times on each of the two days of the Hunger Rehab:

7 AM
10 AM
1 PM
4 PM
7 PM
10 PM

Tips

> Choose a non-working day.

> Keep active to distract yourself from food.

> Be prepared. Get all your ingredients and equipment ready the day before. You really don't want to be in a supermarket surrounded by temptation during your detox.

> Say no to meals out or dinner parties.

> Be positive. Think of this as a clean start.

> Keep it simple – don't cheat.

If you do decide to do the Hunger Rehab, when you get to the end you can go straight on to one of the 14-Day Hunger Types Weight Loss Food Plans. You will know which one is right for you by completing the Hunger Types Quiz on pages 94–7. Good luck!

You will find your personalized Hunger Type weight loss plan on the following pages:

Or you can turn to pages 160–7 to see a chart of all the recipes and their Hunger Types so that you can plan your own weekly menus.

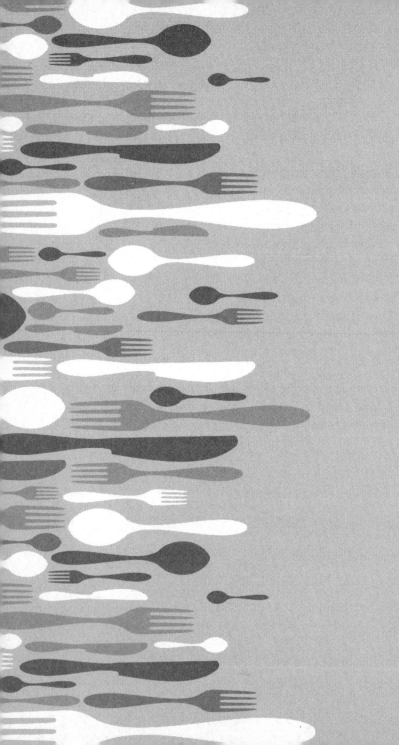

Breakfasts

The Hunger Type Diet starts with getting your breakfast right. By this I mean eating the best food to get all your Hunger Type hormones working properly. And yet this is probably the meal that most people get wrong. How? You're busy, so you grab a couple of slices of toast with jam, or a muffin or a croissant, or you just attach a jump-lead to your brain, aka glug down a strong coffee. But all of these are bound to unbalance your Hunger Type hormones and set off a tsunami of cravings that last for the rest of the day.

The question you should ask yourself first thing before you eat anything is, "Where's the protein?" Not in that slice of toast or that croissant, that's for sure. But protein is important at breakfast in particular, because it sets the pattern for the day. It stabilizes your blood sugar, helps you feel full and is the major raw material for making all your helpful Hunger Type hormones.

The best breakfast protein sources are eggs, yogurt or a smoothie based on whey protein powder. That said, you don't have to do without grains at breakfast. I have included recipes for oatmeal, pancakes, muffins and homemade cereal bars. But you need to portion control your grains to avoid the balance of your breakfast becoming too carby. The sad fact is that just because something is healthy it doesn't mean you can eat your own body weight in it. Once you've had your slice of toast, you need to step away from the loaf.

Many of my clients say they are too busy for breakfast, but that is just as damaging as eating too much or the wrong kind of breakfast, because low blood sugar can result in cravings and weight gain. Others say they aren't hungry, to which I suggest that they think about how much they are eating at night. Our bodies are designed to need fuel when we wake.

A few clients explain to me that when they eat breakfast it makes them hungrier for lunch, so they skip it to help them lose weight. (I used to do that and I weighed 154 pounds—at 5 feet tall.) It's not a very successful strategy. If you think that breakfast makes you hungry, either: (a) it's too high in sugar (including hidden sugar in grains and fruit), which can cause a blood sugar dip later, leading to a surge in sugar cravings; or (b) you didn't eat enough. No one can expect to function properly eating just an apple until lunchtime.

One last point on timing. In my experience working with many weight-loss clients, chaotic eating leads to weight gain, so try to get a good rhythm of meals going from the start. This means eating your breakfast at breakfast time—that is, before 9 AM. This gives you plenty of time to digest it and get naturally hungry for lunch.

BREAKFASTS TO GO

The days when we all sat down to a healthy cooked breakfast are long gone. If you're a working parent, then breakfast is a juggling act—trying to get your offspring to eat something healthy while chasing homework, swimming kits and emptying the washing machine. Many parents I know eat standing up, if at all.

Even those without the responsibility of others to look after in the morning are likely to be in a rush. The combination of long working hours and things like social media—have I checked my facebook yet?—mean that breakfast is grabbed rather then enjoyed.

The popularity of cereal bars, smoothies and instant oatmeal pots proves that for many people the "deskfast", "trainfast" and "busfast" are the norm. But how do you tailor this to suit your Hunger Type and lose weight? Here's how.

Smoothies

There's no doubt that smoothies are fast: whack some fruit into a blender or food processor and *voilà*! Breakfast in a glass. But most smoothies, especially ones you buy ready-squeezed, are high in sugar. Fruits like mango and banana abound. This makes them high GI and not good news for managing Hunger Type hormones.

My Hunger Type smoothies use yogurt or whey protein powder as their base to increase their protein content. You can then afford to add (a little) fruit to sweeten them.

Protein-packed muffins

Muffins are another popular grab-and-go breakfast, but even the so-called "skinny" muffins available from the big coffee chains tend to be stuffed full of refined white flour and sugar, feeding all kinds of cravings.How do you bake a muffin that's not a Hunger Type disaster? Replace some of the flour with whey protein powder, increase the fiber content with bran or add some good fats with seeds. Bake a batch of these and just grab one as you go out the door for a healthy breakfast.

Cereal bars

Shop-bought cereal bars are too high in sugar and many also contain harmful trans fats. Make them yourself for a healthier alternative.

Peanut Butter and Blueberry Smoothie

Many dieters are frightened of peanut butter, because the calorie content is so high. There's no doubt that if you spread it on toast like tile adhesive you'll put on the pounds, but it's full of healthy fats and a little goes a long way, as in this smoothie.

Serves: 2
Preparation time: 5 minutes

¾ cup rolled oats
2 tablespoonss sugar-free smooth peanut butter
2 cups blueberries
½ cup vanilla flavor whey protein powder
4 tablespoons fat-free Greek yogurt
1¾ cups skim milk
2 tablespoons flaxseed

1 Put all the ingredients in a blender or food processor and add 1¼ cups water, then blend until smooth. Serve immediately.

Nutritional analysis per serving
Kcals **371** Protein **22g** Carbohydrate **45g** Fat **12g**

Best for Emotional Hunger, because peanut butter is a source of tryptophan, and we need this to make serotonin, which switches off appetite. Also good for
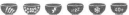

Strawberry and Oatmeal Smoothie

Rolled oats aren't just for oatmeal. They make a worthy addition to a breakfast smoothie, adding healthy fiber and making it more filling.

Serves: 2
Preparation time: 5 minutes

½ cup rolled oats
2 cups fat-free Greek yogurt
scant 1 cup skim milk
2 cups fresh or frozen strawberries
2 teaspoons agave syrup

1 Put all the ingredients into a blender or food processor and blend until smooth. Serve the smoothie immediately.

Nutritional analysis per serving
Kcals **341** Protein **26g** Carbohydrate **51g** Fat **3g**

Best for Anxious Hunger, because oats are a source of glutamic acid, which we need to make the anti-anxiety brain hormone GABA. Also good for

Chocolate and Cherry Smoothie

Although a bar of chocolate is no one's idea of a weight-loss breakfast, using chocolate-flavored whey protein in a smoothie satisfies chocolate cravings in a GI-friendly way.

Serves: 2
Preparation time: 10 minutes

Heaping 1 cup fresh cherries, pitted, or frozen cherries
⅔ cup chocolate flavor whey protein powder
2 tablespoons stevia-based granulated sweetener
1½ tablespoons flaxseed

1 Put all the ingredients in a blender or food processor and add 3 cups water, then blend until smooth. Serve the smoothie immediately.

Nutritional analysis per serving
Kcals **357** Protein **56g** Carbohydrate **33g** Fat **10g**

Best for Cravings Hunger, because cherries are a rich source of vitamin C, which is an important co-factor in the production of dopamine, a key hormone that controls cravings. Also good for

Gingerbread Muffins

I love gingerbread, but even if those little people are iced with a smile, they aren't kind to your wobbly bits. These muffins have the same spicy flavor, but contain much less sugar.

Makes: 6
Preparation time: 10 minutes
Baking time: 30 minutes, plus cooling

1¾ cups whole-wheat flour
2 teaspoons baking powder
2 teaspoons ground ginger
⅓ cup vanilla flavor whey protein powder

1 tablespoon poppy seeds
½ cup granola sweetened with agave syrup (from health-food stores)
15 dried pitted dates, chopped
Heaping ⅔ cup skim milk
Generous ⅓ cup agave syrup
2 eggs
3 tablespoons canola oil

1 Preheat the oven to 350°F. Line a muffin pan with six paper cases. Sift the flour, baking powder, ginger and protein powder into a large bowl. Stir in the poppy seeds, all but 6 teaspoons of the granola and the chopped dates.
2 In another bowl, beat the milk with the agave syrup, eggs and oil, then pour this mixture into the dry ingredients. Stir gently with a wooden spoon until just combined.
3 Fill the muffin cases, sprinkle 1 teaspoon of granola over the top of each one and bake for 25–30 minutes until golden and firm to the touch. Remove from the pan and leave on a wire rack to cool completely before serving.

Nutritional analysis per muffin
Kcals **356** Protein **15g** Carbohydrate **52g** Fat **12g**

 Best for 40+ Hunger, because the natural oils found in seeds are vital for making cell membranes permeable. This can improve the action of sex hormones, helping to balance them and increase weight loss if you are 40+.
Also good for

Bran and Berry Muffins

Oat bran might look like the stuff with which you line a hamster's cage, but it is fantastically high in fiber and low in calories. It bulks out these muffins so that they keep you satisfied until lunchtime.

Makes: 6
Preparation time: 10 minutes
Baking time: 25 minutes, plus cooling

Generous ¾ cup whole-wheat flour
1 teaspoon baking powder
½ teaspoon baking soda
⅓ cup berry flavor whey protein powder
1 tablespoon oat bran

⅓ cup stevia-based granulated sweetener
2 eggs
Heaping ⅓ cup fat-free Greek yogurt
½ cup canola oil
2 teaspoons agave syrup
1 teaspoon vanilla extract
¾ cup fresh strawberries, hulled and finely chopped

1 Preheat the oven to 350°F. Line a muffin pan with six paper cases. Sift the flour, baking powder, baking soda and protein powder into a large bowl. Stir in the bran and sweetener.

2 In another bowl, beat the eggs with the yogurt, oil, agave syrup and vanilla extract, then pour this mixture into the dry ingredients. Add the strawberries and stir gently with a wooden spoon until just combined.

3 Fill the muffin cases and bake for 20–25 minutes until golden brown. Remove the muffins from the pan and leave on a wire rack to cool completely before serving.

Nutritional analysis per muffin
Kcals **290** Protein **13g** Carbohydrate **29g** Fat **22g**

Best for Stress Hunger, because oat bran is rich in B vitamins, which support adrenal function and help you to deal with stress. Boosting B vitamins can give you more energy and reduce stress-related overeating.
Also good for

Surprise Chocolate Muffins

The surprise comes from what's in them—beets. You can't taste it, but it increases the nutrient content and helps keep the muffins moist. You can buy beets ready-cooked in small vacuum packs for convenience. Don't buy the ones in vinegar though, as the muffins really will taste surprising!

Makes: 6
Preparation time: 10 minutes
Baking time: 25 minutes, plus cooling

Scant ½ cup whole-wheat flour
1 teaspoon baking powder
½ cup cocoa powder
⅓ cup chocolate flavor whey protein powder
⅓ cup stevia-based granulated sweetener
2 eggs
½ cup canola oil
1 cup cooked grated beets
⅔ cup skim milk

1 Preheat the oven to 375°F. Line a muffin pan with six paper cases. Sift the flour, baking powder, cocoa powder and protein powder into a large bowl. Stir in the sweetener.
2 In another bowl, beat the eggs with the oil and stir in the beets, then pour this mixture into the dry ingredients. Stir gently with a wooden spoon until just combined.
3 Fill the muffin cases and bake for 20–25 minutes until golden brown. Remove the muffins from the pan and leave on a wire rack to cool completely before serving.

Nutritional analysis per muffin
Kcals **280** Protein **13g** Carbohydrate **11g** Fat **24g**

Best for Tired Hunger, because beet contains the mineral magnesium. Sometimes called nature's tranquillizer, magnesium is a natural muscle relaxant, thereby helping to aid sleep. Good sleep reduces the appetite. Also good for 🥣 🥣 🥣

Peanut Breakfast Bars

These bars are low in sugar, as they're sweetened with the natural low-GI sweetener, agave syrup. It looks a bit like honey, but it is made from a cactus—and it tastes better than that sounds!

Makes: 6
Preparation time: 15 minutes, plus 3 hours chiling

Scant ¼ cup coconut oil
3 tablespoons agave syrup
1 tablespoon sugar-free smooth
  peanut butter
½ cup rolled oats
1½ cups oat bran
2 cups puffed rice
1 tablespoon pumpkin seeds
Heaping ½ cup shredded coconut
⅓ cup peanut-butter flavor whey
  protein powder

1 Put the coconut oil in a small saucepan and add the agave syrup and peanut butter. Heat over low heat, stirring occasionally, until melted and combined.
2 Meanwhile, put all the dry ingredients in a bowl and mix together well.
3 Pour the oil mixture into the dry ingredients and stir to combine. Press into a 12 × 9-inch baking pan and chill in the fridge for 3 hours or until set. Cut into 6 bars before serving. Store in the fridge for up to 7 days.

Nutritional analysis per bar
Kcals **315** Protein **13g** Carbohydrate **32g** Fat **18g**

 Best for Winter-Blues Hunger, because the coconut oil supports thyroid function, which is the gland that controls metabolic rate. A sub-optimal thyroid can make you feel tired and low, two important symptoms of SAD. Also good for

Oat and Almond Power Balls

Strictly speaking, these are balls not bars, but the principle is the same – make in advance and then throw one in a bag for a moveable breakfast.

Makes: 12 (2 balls per serving)
Preparation time: 10 minutes, plus 3 hours chiling

4 tablespoons almond butter
2 tablespoons coconut oil
2 tablespoons agave syrup

1 cup vanilla flavor whey protein powder
2 tablespoons ground flaxseed
4 tablespoons rolled oats
1 tablespoon apple juice, plus extra if needed
2 tablespoons ground almonds

1 Put the almond butter, coconut oil and agave syrup in a large bowl and stir to combine using a wooden spoon. Stir in the protein powder, flaxseed and oats until well-combined. Add as much of the apple juice as you need to make a dough.

2 Divide the mixture into 12 and roll into balls. Put the almonds in a shallow bowl and add the balls two at a time, then roll them in the ground almonds until coated. Put into the fridge to chill for 3 hours, or until they have firmed up, before serving.

Nutritional analysis per 2-ball serving
Kcals **271** Protein **25g** Carbohydrate **16g** Fat **17g**

Best for Anxious Hunger, because almonds and oats are both sources of glutamic acid, which our bodies need to make the calming neurotransmitter GABA. Coconut oil contains a type of fat called medium-chain triglycerides (MCTs), which is used for energy in your body, rather than fat storage, so coconut oil helps weight loss. Also good for

Quinoa Crunch Bars

For those who haven't heard of quinoa, it's a grain used all across Central and South America. Higher in protein than rice or wheat, it makes these bars better at keeping your blood sugar and hunger hormones stable.

Makes: 6
Preparation time: 10 minutes
Baking time: 20 minutes, plus cooling

1½ cups quinoa flakes
½ cup rolled oats
⅓ cup stevia-based granulated sweetener

2 tablespoons ground flaxseed
½ cup chocolate flavor whey protein powder
2 tablespoons cocoa powder
1 tablespoon chopped hazelnuts
scant ½ cup coconut oil, melted
4 tablespoons agave syrup

1 Preheat the oven to 375°F. Line a 12 × 9-inch baking pan with baking parchment. Put all the ingredients in a large bowl and stir well to combine, using a wooden spoon.
2 Tip the mixture into the prepared pan and use your hands to press it down evenly. Bake for 20 minutes or until golden brown. Remove from the pan and leave on a wire rack to cool completely. Cut into 6 bars before serving.

Nutritional analysis per serving
Kcals **368** Protein **15g** Carbohydrate **30g** Fat **25g**

 Best for Cravings Hunger, because cocoa powder contains an amino acid called tyrosine, which we need to make the anti-craving hormone dopamine. Also good for

WORKDAY BREAKFASTS

If you've got a bit more time on a work day, but not that much, you may be able to squeeze in a sit-down-at-the-table breakfast. We're not talking napkins and silverware here, just a healthy meal. It's a worthwhile investment, as starting your day the right way puts you in the best frame of mind for the rest of the day.

Oatmeal

Many of my weight-loss clients love oatmeal. Actually, that is an understatement. They really love oatmeal. They eat big bowls of the stuff, topped with banana and honey in the belief that they are treating their bodies like temples. It's funny how they're not getting any less hungry or any slimmer. Oatmeal is wonderfully comforting and, if you're running a marathon later in the day, great fuel. But it's not a diet food, at least not if you load it up with sugary fruits and more sugar (honey is sugar, after all), and then eat it from a bowl the size of a trash can lid.

Still, with a bit of tweaking, I've come up with some oatmeal ideas that are genuinely good for your Hunger Type hormones and your waistline. All use proper steel-cut oats —also called pinhead oatmeal or coarse oatmeal—which takes longer to cook but is far better for you. If you top it with yogurt, or stir in some very low-fat cottage cheese, this helps to tip the ratio away from carbs to protein even more.

Some people love plain oatmeal, but others find it a big yawn. The problem is, as soon as you start adding toppings, such as honey or jam, you're turning a healthy breakfast into a sugar bomb. Even slicing a banana on top can be blood sugar disrupting. The answer is to make your own super-healthy oatmeal stir-ins.

Alternative-grain oatmeals You don't have to make oatmeal from oats. You can also use lots of other grains to add variety and to extend the range of nutrients you're getting.

Toast

Although toast is convenient, there are two problems with it. First, the bread tends to be made of refined flour; and second, the toppings, such as jam, add more sugar. The way around this is to bake your own bread from grains whose carbs are slower releasing (and it's easier than it sounds) and also to make sure you combine your bread or toast with protein, such as eggs, lean bacon or smoked salmon and so on. I've given two bread recipes here, but you will also find more later in the book.

Toast with what? What could be better than butter to top toasted homemade bread? Other butters, of course. You'll find a selection of toast toppings here.

Eggs

Nourishing eggs are by far the best Hunger Type breakfast. High in protein and containing essential fats, vitamins and minerals, they are fantastic for managing hunger pangs (of all kinds) throughout the day. Eggs also contain the nutrient choline, which helps with brain focus and therefore could help you stick to a diet. You probably find them a giant pain to get ready in the morning, but they don't necessarily have to be. Eggs cook quickly, so they can be a convenient, and a healthy, start to the day.

Homemade Microwave Oatmeal

If you are a fan of those microwave oatmeal pouches, here's a make-your-own recipe. The key is to batch cook (Sunday is a good day to do this), then portion the oatmeal into individual microwaveable servings for reheating each morning. You can even take a daily portion with you to work and stick it in the microwave there. You'll need seven wide-mouthed 2-cup preserving jars, such as Mason jars, so that you can eat the oatmeal from the jar and there will be enough space at the top to add a topping.

Makes: 7 (1 week's breakfasts)
Preparation time: 10 minutes, plus sterilizing the jars and 2 hours cooling
Cooking time: 5 minutes, plus cooling and 3 minutes reheating in a microwave

scant 4¾ cups steel-cut oats (pinhead oats or coarse oatmeal)
4 cups skim milk
a large pinch of sea salt

1 First, sterilize seven wide-mouthed 2-cup Mason jars with screw-top lids. Wash the jars in hot soapy water, rinse and leave them to dry on the shelves in your oven set to 200°F. When dry, turn off the oven and leave the jars inside to cool. Remove the jars, being careful not to touch the insides.
2 Put the oats in a large saucepan and add the milk and salt. Bring to a boil over medium-high heat, then reduce the heat and simmer for 3 minutes.
3 Remove from the heat and allow to cool slightly before ladling into the jars. Leave the jars to stand for 2 hours or until they cool (the oatmeal will continue to cook in the jars), then screw on the lids and store in the fridge.
4 The next morning, remove the lid, then stir the oatmeal and put the jar in the microwave for 2–3 minutes on full power until the oatmeal is heated through. You can then add flavored stir-ins (see pages 202–6).

Nutritional analysis per serving
Kcals **378** Protein **12g** Carbohydrate **65g** Fat **8g**

 Best for Hedonistic Hunger. Oats will help you feel full. They are high in resistant starch, which has been shown to assist weight loss, as it actually helps the body to burn fat. Also good for 🥣 🥣 🥣 🥣 🥣 🥣 🥣 🥣 🥣

Overnight Slow-Cooker Raisin Oatmeal

If even putting something in a microwave is too much trouble, what about waking up to your oatmeal already made and piping hot? With this recipe, you cook the oatmeal overnight in a slow cooker. It's the oatmeal equivalent of an automatic tea maker.

Serves: 2
Preparation time: 5 minutes
Cooking time: 10 hours

1¼ cups steel-cut oats (pinhead oats or coarse oatmeal)
½ cup raisins
a pinch of ground cinnamon
a pinch of ground ginger
a pinch of ground cloves
a pinch of grated nutmeg
2 teaspoons stevia-based granulated sweetener
1–2 drops vanilla extract, to taste
a pinch of sea salt

To serve
1 tablespoon very low-fat cottage cheese
1 teaspoon orange zest

1 The night before, put all the ingredients in the slow cooker, add 1¼ cups water and stir to combine. Set the cooker to Low, put the lid on and leave for 8–10 hours.
2 In the morning, give it a good stir to get rid of any skin and scrape down the sides. You may need to add a little more water, then stir in the cottage cheese, pour into bowls and top with orange zest. Serve.

Nutritional analysis per serving
Kcals **386** Protein **10g** Carbohydrate **75g** Fat **7g**

Best for Emotional Hunger, because raisins are a concentrated source of sugar, and although this is bad for weight loss in large quantities, small doses of sugar from raisins can help to boost the appetite-suppressant hormone serotonin. Also good for 🥣 🥣 🥣

Apple and Vanilla Sauce

Stewed apple is a wonderfully comforting food. Here, I've substituted the usual abundance of sugar for stevia, a lower-calorie and lower-GI natural sweetener.

Serves: 6
Preparation time: 10 minutes, plus making the oatmeal to serve
Cooking time: 40 minutes, plus 5 minutes cooling

scant ½ cup stevia-based granulated sweetener
1 vanilla bean, split lengthwise
fat-free Greek yogurt and oatmeal, to serve

2 tablespoons unsalted butter
1lb 10oz eating apples, peeled, cored and chopped

1 Melt the butter in a saucepan over low heat, add the remaining ingredients and cook for 30–40 minutes until the apple has broken down and formed a thick sauce. Remove the vanilla bean and leave the apple to cool slightly.
2 Pour the apple into a blender or food processor and blend until smooth. Once the oatmeal is reheated in the microwave, add 2 tablespoons yogurt per serving and top with a serving of the sauce.

Tip: Freeze this sauce in an ice-cube tray, then pop out the cubes and store them in a freezer bag so that you have a steady supply of sauce already divided into portions.

Nutritional information per stir-in serving (in addition to the oatmeal)
Kcals **87** Protein **0.3g** Carbohydrate **10g** Fat **4g**

Best for Hedonistic Hunger, because apples are high in a type of fiber called pectin, which swells in the digestive tract to help you feel full. Also good for 🥣 🥣 🥣

Spiced Pear and Prune Compote

Compotes have more texture than fruit sauces, so they don't freeze as well, but this compote can be kept in a jar in the fridge for up to one week.

Serves: 6
Preparation time: 15 minutes, plus making the oatmeal to serve
Cooking time: 12 minutes, plus overnight infusing

1lb 5oz ripe pears, peeled, cored and cut in half
1 vanilla bean, split lengthwise
scant ½ cup stevia-based granulated sweetener
1 cinnamon stick
4 cloves
zest of 1 orange
zest and juice of 1 lemon
¾ cup chopped pitted prunes
fat-free Greek yogurt and oatmeal, to serve

1 Lay the pear halves over the base of a medium saucepan. Scrape out the seeds from the vanilla bean and add them to the pan. Cover with water and heat over medium-high heat. Add the sweetener, spices, orange and lemon zests and the lemon juice. Bring to a boil, then reduce the heat, cover and simmer for 10 minutes or until the pears are tender.
2 Pour off half the syrup into a bowl and add the prunes. Leave the pears in the remaining syrup to infuse overnight. The next morning, cut the pears into smaller chunks. Add them and their syrup to the prunes and stir to combine. Once the oatmeal is reheated in the microwave, serve the fruit on top with 2 tablespoons yogurt per serving.

Nutritional information per serving (in addition to the oatmeal)
Kcals **84** Protein **2g** Carbohydrate **16g** Fat **0.3g**

Best for 40+ Hunger. Cinnamon is a spice with proven blood sugar-regulation properties, important particularly as you get older. Stabilizing blood sugar can reduce fat storage and sugar cravings. Also good for

Blueberry Protein Boost

Stirring whey protein into oatmeal is a really quick and easy way to increase the protein content and make a meal more satisfying.

Serves: 2
Preparation time: 2 minutes, plus making the oatmeal to serve

¼ cup vanilla flavor whey protein powder
1 teaspoon stevia-based granulated sweetener
1¼ cups fresh blueberries
oatmeal, to serve

1 Once the oatmeal is reheated in the microwave, stir in the protein powder and the sweetener, then add the berries and serve.

Nutritional information per stir-in serving (in addition to the oatmeal)
Kcals **81** Protein **10g** Carbohydrate **12g** Fat **0.4g**

Best for Tired Hunger. Blueberries are packed with vitamin C. This is a co-factor in the production of the sleep hormone melatonin. Low melatonin is associated with insomnia and increased appetite. Also good for

Green Banana and Walnut Topping

In general, adding bananas to oatmeal is not a good idea unless you're about to go off for a day down a coal mine, up a chimney or doing another hugely physical job. Bananas are usually too sugary for a weight-loss breakfast, but I realize that many people love them, so I've tweaked the usual recipe, using healthier green bananas.

Serves: 2
Preparation time: 2 minutes, plus making the oatmeal to serve
Cooking time: 30 seconds

⅓ cup chopped walnuts
1 teaspoon stevia-based granulated sweetener
1 green (unripe) banana, sliced
oatmeal, to serve

1 Put the walnuts in a small saucepan and toast them over medium-high heat for 30 seconds. Once the oatmeal is reheated in the microwave, stir in the sweetener and top with the nuts and banana slices, then serve.

Nutritional information per stir-in serving (in addition to the oatmeal)
Kcals **126** Protein **1g** Carbohydrate **15g** Fat **9g**

Best for Never-Full Hunger. Green—that is, unripe—bananas have one of the highest contents of resistant starch of any food (4.7g per banana). This has been shown to increase feelings of fullness and reduce calorie intake later in the day. Also good for 🥣 🥣 🥣 🥣 🥣

Chocolate and Chili Melt

....

OK, I'm not suggesting you have this every day, but it is a real treat.

Serves: 2
Preparation time: 5 minutes, plus making the oatmeal to serve

2 tablespoons very low-fat cottage cheese
2 teaspoons ground cinnamon
1 teaspoon ground coriander
2 tablespoons chocolate flavor whey protein powder
⅓ cup grated dark chocolate with chili
dried chili flakes, to taste
oatmeal, to serve

1 Put the cottage cheese in a small bowl and add the cinnamon, coriander and protein powder. Mix together well. Once the oatmeal is reheated in the microwave, stir the cottage cheese mixture into the oatmeal followed by the chocolate. Top with dried chili flakes and serve.

Nutritional information per stir-in serving (in addition to the oatmeal)
Kcals **101** Protein **14g** Carbohydrate **8.6g** Fat **5g**

Best for Winter-Blues Hunger. Chili is a "thermogenic" food—that is, it speeds up metabolism and calorie burning. This could help those who tend to put on weight in winter. After eating it, the rate at which you burn calories just doing everyday things goes up, which is good news for weight loss. Also good for 🥣 🥣 🌙

Super-Seed Barley Oatmeal

Traditionally, in the US, we put barley in soup, but it also makes a very comforting and substantial "oatmeal".

Serves: 2
Preparation time: 10 minutes, plus overnight soaking
Cooking time: 12 minutes

½ cup pearl barley
1 cup rolled oats
⅔ cup skim milk

seeds of 3 cardamom pods
a pinch of sea salt
a pinch of ground cinnamon
2 teaspoons stevia-based granulated sweetener
1 teaspoon each sunflower, pumpkin, flax and sesame seeds, to serve

1 Put the barley and rolled oats in a large bowl and add water to cover generously. Leave overnight to soak. The next morning, drain the grains and put them in a medium saucepan over medium heat. Add the milk and 2 tablespoons water.
2 Grind the cardamom seeds using a mortar and pestle and add them to the pan with the salt and cinnamon. Bring to a boil, then simmer for 5–10 minutes until the barley is soft (add more water if the mixture sticks to the pan). Remove from the heat and add the sweetener. Pour into bowls and top with the seeds to serve.

Nutritional information per serving
Kcals **329** Protein **9g** Carbohydrate **80g** Fat **9g**

Best for Never-Full Hunger. Adding raw seeds to a meal not only increases the fiber content, but if you chew the seeds well you also release their oils, which slow down stomach emptying, keeping you fuller for longer. Also good for 🥣 🥣 🥣 🥣

Almond and Coconut Oatmeal with Raspberry Swirl

Coconut flour is lower in carbs than most other flours, plus it contains medium-chain triglycerides (MCTs), which your body burns for energy rather than storing it on your backside. It absorbs a lot of liquid, so you may want to add water to this if you find it too thick.

Serves: 2
Preparation time: 5 minutes
Cooking time: 10 minutes

scant ⅔ cup skim milk
1 tablespoon rolled oats
¾ cup ground almonds

2 tablespoons coconut flour
a pinch of sea salt
½ cup fresh or frozen raspberries, plus 6 raspberries, to serve
4 teaspoons stevia-based granulated sweetener

1 Heat the milk in a medium saucepan over medium heat. Stir in the oats, almonds, coconut flour and salt. Reduce the heat, cover the pan and simmer for 3–5 minutes until thickened and cooked through, stirring occasionally.
2 Meanwhile, put the raspberries in a saucepan over medium heat for 1–2 minutes until heated through. (Alternatively, put them in a bowl in the microwave for 1 minute.) Mash the raspberries with a fork.
3 Remove the oatmeal from the heat and stir in the sweetener. Pour into bowls and swirl in the raspberry mixture, then serve.

Nutritional information per serving
Kcals 301 Protein 16g Carbohydrate 25g Fat 25g

 Best for Anxious Hunger. Almonds and oats contain glutamic acid, which we need to make the brain hormone GABA. GABA reduces anxiety, so it may help to reduce anxious overeating. Also good for

Quinoa Oatmeal with Rhubarb and Ginger Jam

You can buy quinoa as a grain or as flakes. This recipe uses flakes, as they are quicker to cook and time is of the essence to many of us first thing.

Serves: 2
Preparation time: 10 minutes
Cooking time: 25 minutes, plus cooling

2 cups quinoa flakes
2 teaspoons ground cinnamon
½ cup skim milk

scant 2½ cups peeled rhubarb chunks
¼ cup stevia-based granulated sweetener
1½ inch piece of ginger root, peeled and grated
4 tablespoons fat-free Greek yogurt, to serve

1 Put the quinoa, cinnamon and milk in a medium saucepan over medium-high heat, bring to a boil, then cover and simmer for 7–10 minutes until the grains start to plump up. Turn off the heat and leave to stand for 15 minutes.
2 Meanwhile, put the rhubarb, sweetener and ginger root in another saucepan over medium-high heat and add ½ cup water. Bring to a boil, then reduce the heat and simmer, uncovered, for 10–15 minutes until the rhubarb is soft and the liquid is syrupy.
3 Leave the rhubarb mixture to cool slightly, then pour into a blender or food processor and blend until smooth. Serve the oatmeal with 2 tablespoons yogurt on each serving and a drizzle of the rhubarb jam.

Nutritional information per serving
Kcals **374** Protein **13g** Carbohydrate **68g** Fat **5g**

Best for Tired Hunger. The volatile oils in ginger have been shown to naturally thin the blood, so improving circulation. This could help lift energy thereby reducing overeating driven by tiredness. Also good for 🥣 🥣 🥣 🥣

Quinoa, Almond and Pumpkin Seed Bread

Quinoa is higher in protein than wheat flour and is also gluten-free. Adding the almond and pumpkin bumps up the protein more and adds brain-friendly essential fats. One important note: you might be tempted to leave the psyllium out. Don't. The bread won't work without it. The seeds give a great taste, but add to the calorie count, so you need to slice this bread thinly.

Makes: 1 loaf (15 slices)
Preparation time: 15 minutes, plus 1 hour 20 minutes soaking
Baking time: 1 hour, plus cooling

1 cup ground almonds
2 cups quinoa flakes
1½ cups pumpkin seeds
generous ½ cup sunflower seeds
2 tablespoons chia seeds
2 tablespoons psyllium husk powder, plus extra if needed
2 tablespoons mixed dried herbs
olive oil spray

1 Put the almonds, quinoa flakes and one-third of the pumpkin seeds in a food processor and process until the consistency of flour. Pour into a bowl and stir in the remaining dry ingredients.
2 Gradually add 2 cups water, stirring. Set aside for 1 hour or until all the water is absorbed. If it's still runny, add some more psyllium husk and leave for 20 minutes more to give you a sticky dough.
3 Preheat the oven to 350°F. Spray an 8 x 4 x 2-inch loaf pan with oil, pour in the bread mixture and use a spoon to press it into the corners. Bake for 40 minutes–1 hour until a toothpick pushed into the center comes out clean. Remove from the oven and turn out onto a wire rack to cool completely. Cut in slices to serve.

Nutritional information per slice
Kcals **201** Protein **7g** Carbohydrate **14g** Fat **13g**

Best for PMS Hunger. Chia seeds are a source of zinc, which may help improve leptin resistance, and this can reduce your appetite and help you to lose weight.
Also good for

Rye and Fennel Seed Bread

This is not only a super-healthy bread, but also as rye is a gluten-free grain it requires no kneading, so it is super-quick too.

Makes: 1 loaf (10 slices)
Preparation time: 15 minutes, plus 2¼ hours rising
Baking time: 55 minutes, plus cooling

1 teaspoon fennel seeds, plus 1 tablespoon for rolling
1 teaspoon cumin seeds, plus 1 tablespoon for rolling
seeds of 8 cardamom pods
2¼ teaspoons active dry yeast
4½ cups rye flour, plus extra for dusting
olive oil spray

1 Put the 1 teaspoon fennel and cumin seeds and the cardamom seeds in a dry skillet and toast over low heat for 1–2 minutes until they release their aroma. Set aside to cool. Put the yeast in a small bowl and add 1¼ cups warm water. Leave for 10 minutes until frothy.

2 Put the toasted seeds and the flour into another bowl and mix together, then make a well in the center and pour in the yeast mixture. Use your hands to mix it into a moist dough. Add more water if it feels dry. Transfer the dough onto a lightly floured work surface and mold it into a loaf shape. Spray an 8 x 4 x 2-inch loaf pan with oil. Roll the dough in the extra seeds and slide it into the prepared pan. Cover with plastic wrap and put it in a warm place for 2 hours or until doubled in size.

3 Preheat the oven to 400°F. Remove the plastic wrap and bake the loaf for 45 minutes or until it sounds hollow when you knock it underneath. Remove from the pan and put on a baking sheet. Bake the loaf for 5 minutes to crisp up the crust. Remove from the pan and leave on a wire rack to cool completely. Cut in slices to serve

Nutritional information per slice
Kcals **194** Protein **8g** Carbohydrate **41g** Fat **2g**

Best for Stress Hunger. Rye bread is low GI, which means it can help to stabilize blood sugar. Unstable blood sugar can cause cravings—typical for Stress Hunger—as well as overeating and weight gain. Also good for 🥣 🥣 🥣

Avocado Butter

Avocados are a fantastic food, full of healthy fats that get all your hunger hormones working brilliantly, but they are high in calories. Here, I've mixed avocado with low-fat cream cheese to make a little go a long way.

Serves: 6
Preparation time: 10 minutes

1 ripe avocado, cut in half and pit removed
Generous ⅓ cup low-fat cream cheese
a squeeze of lemon juice
freshly ground black pepper
6 slices of toast, to serve

1 Using a spoon, scoop out the avocado flesh and put it in a medium bowl. Add the remaining ingredients and season to taste with pepper. Using a fork, mix together well. Use one-sixth of the mixture to top 1 slice of toast and serve.

Nutritional information per serving (in addition to the toast):
Kcals **84** Protein **2g** Carbohydrate **2g** Fat **7g**

 Best for Emotional Hunger. Tryptophan, the amino acid from which appetite-suppressant serotonin is made, is found mostly in protein foods. One notable exception is avocados—eating them can reduce appetite. Also good for 🥣 🥣 🥣 🥣 🥣 🥣 🥣

Reduced-Fat Peanut Butter

Peanut butter is great nutritionally, but it's a bit high in calories. By substituting some of the peanuts with chickpeas, you reduce the fat and the calorie count.

Serves: 10
Preparation time: 10 minutes
Cooking time: 5 minutes, plus cooling and chiling

½ teaspoon cornstarch
¼ cup apple juice

½ teaspoon vanilla extract
½ teaspoon ground cinnamon
1½ cups drained and rinsed canned chickpeas
⅔ cup unsalted peanuts
10 slices of toast, to serve

1 Put the cornstarch in a medium saucepan and stir in the apple juice, then add ¾ cup water, the vanilla extract and cinnamon. Bring to a boil over medium heat, stirring frequently, then reduce the heat and simmer for 2 minutes or until thickened. Set aside to cool.
2 Put the chickpeas and peanuts in a blender or food processor. Gradually add the thickened liquid while you blend the mixture until smooth but not runny. Chill in the fridge before serving as a topping for toast.

Nutritional information per serving of topping (in addition to the toast)
Kcals **86** Protein **4g** Carbohydrate **5g** Fat **5g**

 Best for 40+ Hunger, because chickpeas contain weak plant estrogens called phytestrogens. These can help reduce hormonal fat storage, particularly for women over 40. Also good for

Healthier Chocolate and Hazelnut Spread

We all know the famous chocolate and hazelnut spread that many people love—with predictable spare-tire-multiplying results. My version is a healthier alternative.

Serves: 10
Preparation time: 5 minutes
Baking time: 10 minutes

1 cup hazelnuts
generous ⅓ cup agave syrup
1 tablespoon cocoa powder
10 slices of toast, to serve

1 Preheat the oven to 350°F. Spread out the hazelnuts in a roasting pan and bake for 10 minutes, shaking the pan once, until brown all over (do not allow them to burn). Leave to cool, then leave 1 tablespoon aside.
2 Put the remaining nuts into a food processor and process until the consistency of flour. Add the agave syrup and cocoa powder, and continue to process. Once fully combined, start to add water, a little at a time, until the mixture is smooth but not runny. Pour into a jar, top with the reserved toasted nuts and store in the fridge. Serve as a topping for toast.

Nutritional information per serving of topping (in addition to the toast)
Kcals **120** Protein **3g** Carbohydrate **1g** Fat **3g**

Best for Cravings Hunger. Dark chocolate contains the amino acid L-phenylalanine, which has been shown to raise levels of the anti-cravings hormone dopamine. Also good for 🥣 🥣

Omelets-a-Go-Go

I always think that two eggs scrambled is a pretty sad sight, whereas if you make an omelet from them they look much more substantial. Plus, you can put other things in omelets that add flavor and bulk. My favorites are leftover, home-cooked steamed, baked or stir-fried vegetables.

Serves: 2
Preparation time: 5 minutes
Cooking time: 10 minutes

4 eggs
2 egg whites
olive oil spray

1½ cups leftover cooked vegetables (steamed, baked or stir-fried), such as broccoli, leeks or peas
scant ½ cup half-fat grated hard cheese
sea salt and freshly ground black pepper

1 Put the eggs and whites in a bowl and season with salt and pepper. Beat lightly with a fork, then set aside. Put a nonstick skillet over medium-high heat and spray with oil. Add the eggs. As the mixture sets, use a spatula to pull it away from the side of the pan and allow the mixture to run underneath to ensure there is no runny mixture left.
2 Meanwhile, reheat the vegetables in a colander over a pan of boiling water, or in a microwave, for 1–2 minutes. When the top of the omelet is set and the underneath is golden, scatter the vegetables over the omelet. Top with the grated cheese, fold the omelet in half, cut into two and serve.

A COUPLE OF TWISTS ON THE CLASSIC OMELET
Chinese Omelet *Leave out the grated cheese and add a splash of soy sauce and 1 teaspoon grated ginger root to the eggs.*
Thai Omelet *Leave out the grated cheese and add a dash each of reduced-fat coconut milk and fish sauce to the beaten eggs. Dress with soy sauce and fresh chili.*

Nutritional information per serving
Kcals **322** Protein **28g** Carbohydrate **0.5g** Fat **24g**

 Best for 40+ Hunger, because egg yolks contain progesterone, and increasing it might help offset the weight-storage effects of estrogen dominance in both men and women. Also good for 🥣 🥣 🥣 🥣 🥣

Keralan Omelet with Tomato and Green Chili

I discovered this on vacation once and loved it so much I ate it every day for a week. You don't have to go that far, but it definitely kicks the humble egg up a gear.

Serves: 2
Preparation time: 10 minutes
Cooking time: 10 minutes

4 eggs
2 egg whites
a pinch of sea salt

olive oil spray
1 tomato, diced
½ green chili, seeded and finely chopped
2 tablespoons chopped cilantro leaves
a squeeze of lime juice

1 Put the eggs and whites in a bowl. Add the salt and beat lightly with a fork, then set aside. Put a nonstick skillet over medium-high heat and spray with oil, then pour in the eggs. As the mixture sets, use a spatula to pull it away from the side of the pan and allow the mixture to run underneath to ensure there is no runny mixture left.

2 Sprinkle over the tomato and the chili toward the end of cooking. When the top of the omelet is set and the underneath is golden, sprinkle over the cilantro and the lime juice, then serve.

Nutritional information per serving
Kcals **336** Protein **26g** Carbohydrate **1g** Fat **27g**

Best for Cravings Hunger, because eggs are high in protein, which helps balance blood sugar and prevent cravings. Also good for 🥣 🌙 ❄️

Mexican Breakfast Tortilla

If you want something just a bit more substantial than an omelet, and pretty portable too, this omelet in a wrap is ideal.

Serves: 2
Preparation time: 10 minutes
Cooking time: 12 minutes

olive oil spray
2 kale leaves, chopped
1 onion, finely chopped
1 green bell pepper, seeded and finely chopped
1 red bell pepper, seeded and finely chopped
1 zucchini, finely chopped
¼ bird's eye chili, seeded and chopped
scant ½ cup tomato sauce
2 eggs
2 whole-wheat tortillas
sea salt and freshly ground black pepper
chopped cilantro leaves, to serve

1 Put a nonstick skillet over medium-high heat and spray with oil. Add the vegetables, chili and tomato sauce, then season and cook for 5 minutes.
2 Make two wells in the center of the vegetable mixture and spray more oil into them, then add 1 egg into each well. Cover the pan and cook for 3–4 minutes until the eggs are cooked to your liking.
3 Put an egg and some of the tomato mixture in the center of each tortilla, then sprinkle with cilantro, fold up and serve.

Nutritional information per serving
Kcals **228** Protein **15g** Carbohydrate **15g** Fat **11g**

Best for Stress hunger. Kale contains sulfur, which helps liver detoxification of excess hormones including the stress hormone cortisol. This can improve hormone balance and weight loss. Also good for

WEEKEND LIE-IN BREAKFASTS

Many people manage to eat healthily during the week, but then the wheels come off big style at the weekend. Without their normal routine, and with 24-hour access to the fridge, they go mad.

Saturday and Sunday may be the only days of the week when you have the time or inclination to cook a "proper" breakfast, so this section includes recipes for homemade breakfast rolls, pancakes and even a twist on the popular Welsh rarebit.

The trick? It's natural to want to indulge yourself on Saturday and Sunday, so here are some treat breakfasts that are also Hunger Type-hormone friendly.

Pecan Pancakes with Crispy Bacon

Pancakes are the quintessential brunch-style breakfast—include cottage cheese to make them great for your Hunger Type hormones.

Serves: 2
Preparation time: 10 minutes
Cooking time: 15 minutes

2 lean Canadian bacon slices
1 egg, beaten
½ cup skim milk
scant 1 cup whole-wheat flour
1 teaspoon baking powder
a pinch of sea salt

1 tablespoon stevia-based granulated
  sweetener
scant ¼ cup very low-fat cottage
  cheese
olive oil spray

To serve
1 tablespoon agave syrup
2 pecans, chopped

1 Preheat the broiler. Put the bacon on a broiler pan and broil until golden on both sides, turning over once. Meanwhile, put the egg and milk in a small pitcher and beat together well.
2 Sift the flour, baking powder, salt and sweetener into another bowl, then make a well in the center and pour in the egg mixture. Beat with a wooden spoon to create a smooth batter, then stir in the cottage cheese.
3 Put a nonstick skillet over medium-high heat and spray with oil. Drop in spoonfuls of the mixture to thinly coat the base of the pan. Cook for 1 minute or until bubbles start to appear on the surface of the batter, then flip the pancake over using a spatula and cook the other side. Repeat with the remaining batter.
4 Put the agave syrup and pecans in a small saucepan over medium-low heat and gently heat through. Serve the pancakes with the sauce poured over and with the bacon on top.

Nutritional information per serving
Kcals **410** Protein **26g** Carbohydrate **48g** Fat **58g**

Best for Cravings Hunger. Dairy products such as milk and cottage cheese contain calcium, which has been shown to reduce levels of the appetite hormone ghrelin, thereby switching off hunger. Also good for

Coconut Pancakes with Black Forest Drizzle

A really luxurious breakfast that's also good for you.

Serves: 2
Preparation time: 15 minutes
Cooking time: 15 minutes

2 eggs
1–2 drops vanilla extract, to taste
⅓ cup coconut flour
4 teaspoons stevia-based granulated

sweetener
a pinch of sea salt
½ teaspoon baking powder
scant ⅔ cup frozen forest fruits
olive oil spray
fat-free Greek yogurt, to serve

1 Put the eggs and vanilla extract in a small bowl and beat together. Put the flour in another bowl and add the sweetener, salt and baking powder. Mix well, then make a well in the center and pour in the eggs. Beat to make a smooth batter using a wooden spoon. Set aside.
2 Meanwhile, put the forest fruits in a saucepan over medium heat and heat through for 1–2 minutes. (Alternatively, put them in a bowl in the microwave for 1 minute until hot.) Mash the forest fruits with a fork. Add a little water to make the purée into a sauce.
3 Put a nonstick skillet over medium-high heat and spray with oil.
Drop in spoonfuls of the mixture to thinly coat the base of the pan. Cook for 1–2 minutes until bubbles start to appear on the surface of the batter, then flip the pancake over using a spatula and cook the other side. Repeat with the remaining batter. Serve the pancakes with 2 tablespoons Greek yogurt per serving and drizzled with the forest fruits sauce.

Nutritional information per serving
Kcals **333** Protein **16g** Carbohydrate **12g** Fat **23g**

Best for Cravings Hunger. Berries are one of the few fruit categories that have a low GI, meaning that they don't upset blood sugar and cause cravings later. Also good for

Mushroom Rarebit

Traditional Welsh Rarebit, aka cheese on toast, is very high in carbs. Substituting mushrooms for the toast is much healthier. This recipe makes enough cheese mixture for two servings, but you can freeze the extra serving for another day if you are making it for one.

Serves: 2
Preparation time: 15 minutes
Cooking time: 20 minutes, plus cooling

scant ¼ cup skim milk
heaping 1 cup freshly grated Parmesan cheese
1 cup grated reduced-fat Cheddar cheese
1 tablespoon fresh whole-wheat bread crumbs
1 tablespoon all-purpose flour
1 egg yolk
a pinch of English mustard powder
olive oil spray
6 large portobello mushrooms, stalks removed
sea salt and freshly ground black pepper

1 Put the milk in a medium saucepan and add both cheeses. Heat over medium heat, stirring, until the cheese has melted. Sprinkle over the bread crumbs and flour, then stir in and cook for 2–3 minutes until thickened, stirring continuously. Remove from the heat and leave to cool slightly, then stir in the egg yolk and mustard powder, and season with salt and pepper. Cool, then transfer to the fridge until ready to use.

2 Preheat the oven to 400°F. Spray an ovenproof dish with oil and then put the mushrooms, gill-side up, in the dish. Spoon half the cheese mixture into the mushroom cups. Bake for 10–15 minutes until the cheese is golden and bubbling, then serve.

Nutritional information per serving
Kcals **413** Protein **46g** Carbohydrate **7g** Fat **22g**

Best for Winter-Blues Hunger. Eggs and milk are both excellent sources of vitamin D. In summer we can get this from the sunshine, but in winter a lack of vitamin D is associated with depression and overeating. Also good for 🍽 🌙 40+

Overnight Breakfast Rolls with Scrambled Eggs and Smoked Salmon

....

These rolls involve making a no-knead mixture the night before and leaving it overnight in the fridge to bake the next day. Easy-peasy. If there is only one or two of you, freeze the extra dough and reduce the eggs and salmon.

Serves: 4
Preparation time: 5 minutes, plus overnight rising
Baking time: 30 minutes, plus cooling

1 ¼ teaspoons active dry yeast
a pinch of sea salt
1¾ cups whole-wheat flour
¼ cup pumpkin seeds

For the scrambled eggs
4 eggs
7oz smoked salmon, cut into strips
olive oil spray
sea salt and freshly ground black pepper
2 teaspoons chopped chives, to serve

1 The night before, put all the bread ingredients in a bowl and add 1 scant cup water. Mix together well—it will seem very wet. Cover with plastic wrap and chill overnight in the fridge.

2 Next morning, preheat the oven to 425°F. Line a baking sheet with parchment paper. Drop 4 heaps of the dough onto the pan, making them as high as you can and leaving space in between (they will look quite flat). Bake for 20 minutes until lightly browned and they sound hollow when tapped underneath. Leave on a wire rack to cool completely.

3 Put the eggs in a bowl and season with salt and pepper. Beat lightly with a fork, then add the salmon.

4 Spray a nonstick skillet with oil, then put it over medium heat and add the egg mixture. Cook, stirring with a wooden spoon, so that the eggs scramble to make soft curds. When almost completely set, remove from the heat, cover with a lid and leave for 2 minutes. Serve the rolls with the eggs sprinkled with chopped chives.

Nutritional information per serving
Kcals **412** Protein **16g** Carbohydrate **41g** Fat **4g**

Best for Winter-Blues Hunger. A deficiency of omega-3 fats such as those found in oily fish can be a factor in depressed overeating and SAD. Boosting these fats can therefore help weight loss. Also good for

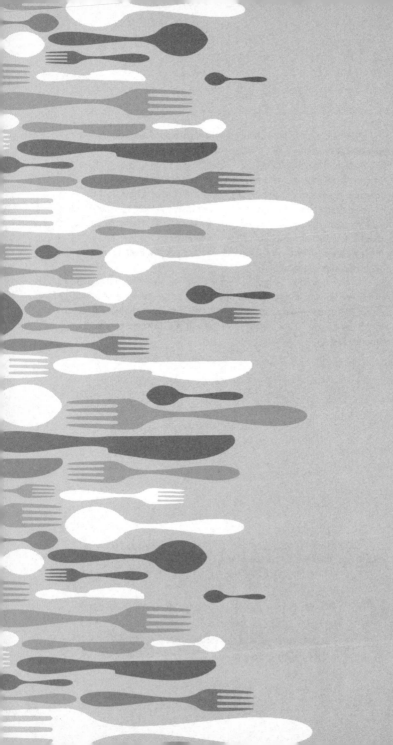

Lunches

"Fail to plan and plan to fail", or as gung-ho personal trainers tend to say, anyway. While much of the "go, go, go!" element of PT-speak is highly irritating, this bit is, I'm afraid, true. Preparation makes dieting much easier, especially for lunchtimes, which may have to be eaten away from home in an office lunchroom, a café, diner, or even the car. For this reason, I've included a number of meals in this section that can be packed. My Hunger Type salads, soups and sandwiches are all designed to provide the right balance of lean protein, good carbs and healthy fats to help all Hunger Types lose weight. Plus, look out for the special recipes tailored specifically for your Hunger Type.

SALADS

Salad is the stereotypical diet food. Indeed, in my last book (*The Serotonin Revolution: The Low-Carb Diet that Won't Make You Crazy*), I didn't include them for this reason. I wanted to offer something different. However, there is no doubt that the sheer volume of salad you can eat for very few calories makes them useful for weight loss.

Plus, there is such a variety of tastes and textures you can create. There is an enormous variety of leaves available, from butter lettuce to iceberg, through arugula and baby spinach and who knows how many more. You can add in tomatoes, salad onions and raw veggies, like grated carrot or zucchini. Then there are all the dressings you can try out. Even if you think you hate salads, there has to be one you will like.

The trouble with many store-bought lunch salads is that they contain white pasta, which will unbalance your blood sugar and leave you feeling sleepy in the afternoon, craving sugar. My Hunger Type salads are filling, healthy and packable. If you are going to transport them, put the wettest ingredients at the bottom of your plastic box and take your dressing separately to prevent the lettuce wilting.

Cheat's Chicken Caesar Salad

If there's one thing that accounts for the normally astronomical calorie content of Caesar salad, it's the dressing. I've lightened this version by reducing the amount of Parmesan cheese, but it still tastes great.

Serves: 2
Preparation time: 15 minutes
Cooking time: 3 minutes, plus cooling

2 tablespoons pumpkin seeds
1 romaine lettuce, separated into leaves
12 cherry tomatoes
7oz cooked skinless chicken breast, sliced

For the Caesar dressing
1 egg yolk
4 canned anchovies, drained on paper towels
1 garlic clove, crushed
juice of ½ lemon
1 teaspoon Dijon mustard
⅓ cup freshly grated Parmesan cheese
1 tablespoon olive oil
1 tablespoon white wine vinegar
freshly ground black pepper

1 Put the pumpkin seeds in a nonstick skillet and dry-fry for 2–3 minutes until they swell slightly, but do not burn. Leave to cool.
2 Put the lettuce leaves and tomatoes on two plates and top with the chicken and pumpkin seeds.
3 Put the dressing ingredients into a blender or food processor and blend until smooth. Dress the salad just before serving.

Nutritional information per serving
Kcals **381** Protein **45g** Carbohydrate **6g** Fat **18g**

Best for Emotional Hunger. Although turkey is well known for being high in the amino acid tryptophan, chicken is also a good source. Tryptophan is converted in the body into the appetite-suppressant hormone serotonin. Also good for

Chicken and Green Mango Salad

Normal, ripe mangos are a very sweet fruit that can really upset blood sugar, setting you up for overeating later. Eat them green, however, and they don't have the same effect.

Serves: 2
Preparation time: 15 minutes

2 little gem lettuces, separated into leaves
1 cucumber, sliced
2 carrots, peeled and grated
8oz cooked skinless chicken breast, sliced
1 green mango, peeled, pitted and cut into matchsticks

For the chili dressing
juice of 2 limes
1 small red chili, seeded and finely chopped
2 tablespoons Thai fish sauce
1 tablespoon stevia-based granulated sweetener
1 teaspoon sesame oil
2 shallots, finely chopped

1 Put the salad ingredients on two plates. Top with the chicken and mango.
2 Put the dressing ingredients in a screw-topped jar and shake well. Dress the salad just before serving.

Tip: This dressing tastes better if you let the flavor develop over 4 hours or more.

Nutritional information per serving
Kcals **330** Protein **32g** Carbohydrate **49g** Fat **6g**

Best for Tired Hunger. Mango is a good source of energy-giving iron. This can help weight loss by giving you energy to exercise and preventing you using high-calorie snacks to offset tiredness. Also good for 🌀 🥣 ❄️

Turkey and Broccoli Salad with Gremolata

Gremolata is an Italian herby, lemony topping that works well for salad, but you can also sprinkle it over meat or fish.

Serves: 2
Preparation time: 15 minutes
Cooking time: 5 minutes

8oz broccoli florets
1 romaine lettuce, separated into leaves
1 bunch watercress
8 pitted black olives, chopped

8oz cooked skinless turkey breast, sliced
a pinch of dried chili flakes

For the gremolata
1 garlic clove, crushed
zest and juice of 1 lemon
1 bunch each of parsley and arugula
2 tablespoons extra virgin olive oil

1 Put the broccoli in a steamer over boiling water and cook for 5 minutes or until crisp-tender. Remove from the pan and refresh in cold water to cool.
2 Put the broccoli and salad ingredients on two plates. Top with the olives and turkey, and sprinkle with chili flakes.
3 Put the gremolata ingredients into a blender or food processor and pulse to create a sauce. Dress the salad just before serving.

Nutritional information per serving
Kcals **339** Protein **36g** Carbohydrate **6g** Fat **19g**

 Best for PMS Hunger. Broccoli, like all the brassica vegetables (cauliflower, cabbage, Brussels sprouts), contains sulfur. Although you shouldn't eat these vegetables raw, because they slow down the thyroid and can be a factor in weight gain, when cooked the sulfur supports liver function, which assists hormone balance and weight loss. Also good for

Salmon and Avocado Salad with Wasabi Vinaigrette

Wasabi is the hot green horseradish you find in Japanese restaurants. It's very hot, so use with care!

Serves: 2
Preparation time: 15 minutes
Cooking time: 10 minutes, plus cooling

olive oil spray
2 salmon fillets, 4 oz each
2 heads of red Belgian endive, separated into leaves
2 handfuls of baby spinach leaves

12 cherry tomatoes
1 large, ripe avocado, peeled, pitted and sliced

For the wasabi vinaigrette
juice of 2 limes
2 tablespoons extra-virgin olive oil
2 teaspoons wasabi
1 teaspoon agave syrup

1 Preheat the broiler and spray the broiler pan with oil. Put the salmon on the broiler pan, skin-side up, and spray with oil. Cook for 4 minutes on each side or until the fish is opaque and firm to the touch. Leave to cool.
2 Put the salad ingredients, except the avocado, on two plates. Top with the salmon and avocado.
3 Put the dressing ingredients into a screw-topped jar and shake gently. Dress the salad just before serving.

Tip: If you're packing this one, put the avocado in with the dressing to stop it turning brown.

Nutritional information per serving
Kcals **393** Protein **25g** Carbohydrate **18g** Fat **28g**

Best for 40+ Hunger. Spinach contains both energy-boosting iron and relaxing magnesium, so it may help to regulate your natural circadian rhythm or wake–sleep cycle, which can be a particular problem after 40. An upset 24-hour cycle can lead to overeating. Also good for 🍲 🌙 ❄️

Mackerel Salad with Creamy Horseradish Dressing

Smoked mackerel is a great way to get your Hunger Type hormone-friendly omega-3 fats. Plus, it's already cooked, so there's no need to stink your house out cooking fish. Still, it's calorie dense, so a little goes a long way. Make sure to cut one fillet into two portions.

Serves: 2
Preparation time: 15 minutes

1 romaine lettuce, separated into leaves
2 celery stalks, chopped
1 red onion, thinly sliced
4 oz smoked mackerel fillet, skin removed, cut into 2 pieces

For the horseradish dressing
4 tablespoons fat-free Greek yogurt
1 teaspoon stevia-based granulated sweetener
2 teaspoons creamed horseradish
a squeeze of lemon juice

1 Put the salad ingredients on two plates and top with the mackerel.
2 Put the dressing ingredients in a bowl and stir together to combine. Dress the salad just before serving.

Nutritional information per serving
Kcals **421** Protein **24g** Carbohydrate **7g** Fat **32g**

Best for Anxious Hunger. Many people overeat when they are anxious. This can be improved by eating mackerel, because it is a source of glutamic acid, which we need to make the anti-anxiety neurotransmitter GABA. Also good for

Asian Slaw with Shrimp

I love Vietnamese salads, because they taste so fresh and healthy, but they often contain a whack of palm sugar. I've just swapped this for stevia to make it even more Hunger Type compatible.

Serves: 2
Preparation time: 15 minutes

6½ cups (14 oz) shredded green cabbage
6½ cups (14 oz) shredded red cabbage
12 radishes, finely sliced
2 scant cups bean sprouts
2 cups cooked peeled shrimp
2 tablespoons chopped salted peanuts
2 tablespoons chopped cilantro leaves

For the Asian dressing
zest and juice of 1 lime
2 teaspoons stevia-based granulated sweetener
2 teaspoons sesame oil
½ red chili, seeded and chopped
¾-inch piece of ginger root, peeled and grated

1 Put both types of cabbage, the radishes and bean sprouts on two plates. Top with the shrimp and sprinkle over the peanuts and cilantro.
2 Put the dressing ingredients in a screw-topped jar and shake well. Dress the salad just before serving.

Nutritional information per serving
Kcals **346** Protein **30g** Carbohydrate **8g** Fat **13g**

 Best for Never-Full Hunger. Peanuts are a ground nut and less nutritious than tree nuts. But, for weight loss, they have an important benefit—they contain tryptophan, which the body uses to make appetite-suppressant serotonin. Also good for 🍲 🍲 🍲

Egg Salad with Spicy Tomato Dressing

Most egg salad sandwiches are a sickly yet bland combination of egg and greasy mayonnaise. This one is lighter and a bit spicy.

Serves: 2
Preparation time: 15 minutes
Cooking time: 10 minutes, plus cooling

4 eggs
½ iceberg lettuce, shredded
scant 1½ cups frozen corn kernels, defrosted
2 carrots, peeled and grated
1 celery stalk, chopped

8 baby plum tomatoes, cut in half
2 tablespoons chopped mint leaves
2 tablespoons chopped cilantro leaves

For the spicy tomato dressing
2 tablespoons fat-free Greek yogurt
1 teaspoon stevia-based granulated sweetener
1 tablespoon tomato paste
a dash of Tabasco sauce

1 Put the eggs in a pan of boiling water and cook for 10 minutes. Drain the eggs and put them into a bowl of cold water to cool. Peel off the shells and dice the eggs.
2 Put the salad vegetables on two plates. Top with the eggs and sprinkle with the fresh herbs. Put the dressing ingredients in a bowl and stir well to combine. Dress the salad just before serving.

Nutritional information per serving
Kcals **270** Protein **18g** Carbohydrate **13g** Fat **10g**

Best for Winter-Blues Hunger. Many people assume that you can only get omega-3s from fish like salmon, but eggs—especially organic eggs—can also be a good source. Omega-3s help all your hunger hormones to work better – particularly helpful in the colder weather. Also good for

Feta, Walnut and Pomegranate Salad

Feta cheese is made from sheep's milk, not cow's, so those who have a problem with dairy may be able to tolerate it. It's strong, so a little goes a long way.

Serves: 2
Preparation time: 15 minutes

½ pomegranate
⅓ cup chopped walnuts

2 Boston lettuces, separated into leaves
2 cups arugula
1 cucumber, diced
1 red onion, thinly sliced
¾ cup cubed feta cheese

For the dill dressing
2 tablespoons extra virgin olive oil
1 tablespoon red wine vinegar
1 teaspoon stevia-based granulated sweetener
2 tablespoons chopped dill

1 Put the salad ingredients on two plates. Top with the feta cheese.
2 Cut the pomegranate half into quarters and push out the seeds. Discard the pith. Sprinkle the pomegranate seeds and walnuts over the salad.
3 Put the dressing ingredients in a screw-topped jar and shake well. Dress the salad just before serving.

Nutritional information per serving
Kcals **392** Protein **10g** Carbohydrate **12g** Fat **109g**

Best for Cravings Hunger. Walnuts are a source of the amino acid tyrosine, which the body needs to make the cravings-beating hormone dopamine. Also good for 🥣 🥣 🥣

SOUPS

Nourishing soup is a brilliant lunchtime standby. If you make it in advance, you can reheat it in a trice, plus it packs really well. The important thing with Hunger Type soups is that they are meals in themselves, so they all contain a protein source (meat, poultry, fish, beans or tofu). This makes them filling and balances blood sugar in a way that a simple vegetable soup never can.

Soup is especially important for reducing hunger, because research says that it pushes down appetite-stimulating ghrelin levels; for example, if you eat chicken and a glass of water, the water passes straight through the stomach. But if you eat chicken soup, the water in the soup stays in the stomach, adding volume and switching off ghrelin. Too much ghrelin is a big problem for Hedonist Hunger Types (see page 48), so they should really think about eating more soup, but it will help all Hunger Types.

That said, there's nothing so horrible (in my opinion) as watery diet-vegetable soup (does anyone remember Shapers diet soups from the 1980s?). My Hunger Type soups are a million miles from that—thick and comforting, chunky textured, intensely flavored or all three. Many feature beans. I'm not trying to turn you into a knit-your-own-sandals-and-teepee veggie, but beans are great in soups, because when you partly purée the finished result, you get a creamy texture without the need to add thigh-expanding cream.

Soups work best when you make a big batch, so I've made these recipes to serve four. You can eat one portion and then chill or freeze the rest.

Thai Chicken and Mushroom Broth

If you want a super-tasty but also super-low-cal soup, then Asian broths are the way to go. This one has healthy chicken and mushrooms.

Serves: 4
Preparation time: 15 minutes
Cooking time: 10 minutes

4 cups hot chicken bouillon
1 tablespoon Thai red curry paste
1 tablespoon Thai fish sauce
2 teaspoons stevia-based granulated sweetener

zest and juice of 2 limes
2 cups sliced Portobello mushrooms
1 bunch scallions, white and green parts separated, sliced
2½ cups cooked cubed skinless chicken breast

1 Put all the ingredients, except the green parts of the scallions and the chicken, into a large saucepan over medium-high heat. Bring to a boil, then reduce the heat, cover and simmer for 5 minutes.
2 Add the chicken and heat through for 3 minutes. Serve topped with the spring onion greens.

Nutritional information per serving
Kcals **123** Protein **25g** Carbohydrate **3g** Fat **5g**

 Best for Never-Full Hunger. Mushrooms are high in beta glucans, a form of resistant starch, which can help you feel full and so prevent overeating. Also good for

Chinese Pork and Spinach Broth

Are you put off making soup because of the endless chopping and sautéing? Forget it with this one. This is the easiest soup ever!

Serves: 4
Preparation time: 10 minutes
Cooking time: 10 minutes

14oz pork tenderloin, cut into thin strips
4 cups chicken bouillon
2 tablespoons soy sauce

2 teaspoons Chinese five-spice powder
1½-inch piece of ginger root, peeled and cut into matchsticks
1lb baby spinach
1 red chili, seeded and chopped
1 bunch of scallions, sliced

1 Put all the ingredients in a large saucepan over medium heat, cover and bring to a boil, then reduce the heat and simmer gently for 8 minutes or until the pork is cooked. Serve.

Nutritional information per serving
Kcals **168** Protein **23g** Carbohydrate **4g** Fat **10g**

Best for Stress Hunger. People used to think that pork was unhealthy, but lean pork has a similar lean-to-fat profile as turkey, plus it contains iron, zinc and B vitamins. B vitamins are important for weight loss, as they help us deal with stress and so may prevent stress-eating. Also good for 🥣 🥣 🥣

Ouillade

Sometimes you just want a really comforting traditional soup. This French soup combines the deliciously savory taste of ham with sweet turnip and then ups the nutritional input with that vegetable *du jour*, kale.

Serves: 4
Preparation time: 15 minutes, plus overnight soaking
Cooking time: 1 hr 25 minutes, plus cooling

14oz unsmoked ham hock, soaked overnight and drained
¾ cup dried navy beans, soaked overnight and drained
olive oil spray
1 onion, chopped
2 carrots, peeled and chopped
¾ cup diced turnip or rutabaga
4 cups chopped curly kale (from about 5oz kale stalks)
2 garlic cloves, finely chopped
1 tablespoon chopped parsley leaves
freshly ground black pepper

1 Put the ham hock in a saucepan over medium-high heat and cover with 4 cups water. Bring to a boil, then reduce the heat, cover and simmer for 45 minutes, turning the ham over as the liquid reduces. The meat should be falling off the bone.

2 Leave to cool in the liquid, then lift out the ham hock and set aside. Strain the liquid from the ham through a sieve into a pitcher and reserve.

3 While the ham is cooking, put the beans in another saucepan with 2 cups water. Bring to a boil, then reduce the heat, cover and simmer for 45 minutes, removing with a spoon any scum that rises to the surface. Drain in a colander and set aside.

4 Put a large nonstick saucepan over medium heat and spray with oil, then fry the onion for 3–4 minutes until soft. Add the carrots and cook for 5–10 minutes until soft (add some of the ham bouillon if it sticks to the pan). Add 4 cups of the ham bouillon and the turnips, return to a boil, then simmer for 10 minutes.

5 Meanwhile, remove the skin from the ham, then tear the meat into small pieces. Add this, plus the kale and the beans to the soup and simmer for 5 minutes. Remove the pan from the heat, stir in the garlic, parsley and black pepper, and serve.

Nutritional information per serving
Kcals **382** Protein **39g** Carbohydrate **33g** Fat **6g**

Best for 40+ Hunger. Kale is a sulfurous vegetable (like cauliflower and broccoli), which boosts liver detoxification and can improve hormone balance and help weight loss. Also good for 🥣 🥣 🥣 🥣

Hungarian Beef and Beet Soup

Not all red meat is bad for you. Advice that saturated fat in meat was a heart attack waiting to happen is now changing, and free-range meat from animals such as grass-fed beef actually contains super-healthy omega-3 fats too. Plus, red meat gives you a great dollop of highly bio-available iron, which is the most commonly deficient mineral in many of us.

Serves: 4
Preparation time: 20 minutes
Cooking time: 1¾ hours

olive oil spray
14oz stewing beef, cut into small dice
1 onion, chopped
2 garlic cloves, crushed
1 tablespoon paprika

1 teaspoon cumin seeds
3 cups beef bouillon
9oz potatoes, peeled and diced
1 x 14oz can chopped tomatoes
1lb raw beets, unpeeled, trimmed
1 tablespoon chopped dill
2 tablespoons chopped parsley leaves
sea salt and freshly ground black
    pepper

1 Preheat the oven to 400°F. Put a large nonstick saucepan over medium-high heat and spray with oil, then fry the beef in batches to brown it on all sides. Transfer to a plate and set aside.

2 Spray the pan and add the onion. Fry over medium heat for 3–4 minutes to soften, then add the garlic and spices. Cook for 1 minute (add a splash of bouillon if the mixture sticks to the pan). Add the potatoes and stir to coat with the onion mixture. Return the beef to the pan and add the tomatoes and bouillon. Season with salt and pepper. Bring to a boil, then cover and simmer over low heat for 1½ hours or until the beef is tender.

3 Meanwhile, wrap the beets in aluminum foil and bake for 40 minutes. Leave to cool. Peel and cut into ½-inch dice. Add to the soup with the herbs. Serve.

Nutritional information per serving
Kcals **383** Protein **39g** Carbohydrate **28g** Fat **11g**

Best for Cravings Hunger. Beets are great for beating cravings, because they contain folic acid, an essential co-factor that converts tyrosine to the anti-craving brain hormone dopamine. Also good for 🥣 🥣 🥣

Spanish Fish Soup

I love fish soup—but not the kind where you have to scoop out bits of bone (I have a thing about bones), however authentically peasanty that might be. This one features boneless white fish, beans, vegetables and lots of lovely smoked paprika.

Serves: 4
Preparation time: 15 minutes
Cooking time: 30 minutes

olive oil spray
1 onion, chopped
2 garlic cloves, crushed
1 teaspoon paprika
1 teaspoon cayenne pepper
9oz potatoes, peeled and diced

zest and juice of 1 lemon
1 x 14oz can chopped tomatoes
2½ cups vegetable bouillon
1 x 14oz can chickpeas, drained and
 rinsed
1lb cod or pollock fillet, skinned and
 cut into large chunks
1 handful parsley leaves, chopped
sea salt and freshly ground black
 pepper

1 Put a large nonstick saucepan over medium heat and spray with oil, then fry the onion for 3–4 minutes until soft. Add the garlic and spices and fry for another 1 minute.

2 Add the potatoes and stir to coat with the onion mixture, then add the lemon zest and juice, and leave to sizzle for 30 seconds. Add the tomatoes and bouillon, and season with salt and pepper. Bring to a boil, then reduce the heat, cover and simmer for 10–15 minutes until the potatoes are almost cooked.

3 Add the chickpeas and fish, return to a simmer and cook for 8 minutes or until the fish is cooked through. Sprinkle with the parsley and serve.

Nutritional information per serving
Kcals **298** Protein **32g** Carbohydrate **34g** Fat **5g**

Best for 40+ Hunger. Many people don't want to cook oily fish because of the cooking smells, but you can get your hunger hormone-modulating omega-3s another way. Less smelly white fish contains them too, albeit in smaller amounts. Also good for 🥣 🌙 ❄️

Healthy Shrimp Laksa

Laksa is superb, but most recipes are incredibly fattening, because of the combination of rice noodles (they're way off the GI scale) and gallons of coconut milk. This one uses reduced-fat coconut milk and substitutes bean sprouts for the noodles.

Serves: 4
Preparation time: 20 minutes
Cooking time: 15 minutes

14oz large raw shrimp, peeled
olive oil spray
1 tablespoon Thai red curry paste
3 cups vegetable bouillon

1 red bell pepper, seeded and sliced
1¼ lb fresh beansprouts
1¾ cups reduced-fat coconut milk
juice of 1 lime
2 tablespoons stevia-based granulated
sweetener
1 small handful of cilantro leaves,
chopped

1 Make a shallow cut down the center of the curved back of each shrimp. Pull out the black vein with a toothpick or your fingers, then rinse the shrimp thoroughly. Set aside.

2 Put a large nonstick saucepan over medium heat and spray with oil, then fry the curry paste for 1–2 minutes to release its aroma. Add the bouillon, bring to a boil and then add the shrimp. Cover and simmer for 5 minutes or until they are pink.

3 Add the bell pepper and beansprouts, and cook for 2 minutes, then add the coconut milk. Bring back to a boil, then reduce the heat to a simmer and stir in the lime juice and sweetener. Add the cilantro leaves and serve.

Nutritional information per serving
Kcals **203** Protein **27g** Carbohydrate **10g** Fat **15g**

Best for Emotional Hunger. Beansprouts may seem a fairly pointless vegetable, but they are actually a good source of B vitamins, which can give you energy if you're feeling low and prevent you comfort eating. Also good for

Zucchini and White Bean Soup

This is a really pretty soup, and it's also substantial. It's simple to make, with a reassuringly short ingredients list.

Serves: 4
Preparation time: 15 minutes, plus overnight soaking
Cooking time: 35 minutes

olive oil spray
1 onion, chopped
1 garlic clove, crushed
1¾ cups dried navy beans, soaked overnight and drained

½ leek, cut in half and sliced
2 zucchinis, cut lengthwise, seeded and diced
4 cups vegetable bouillon
generous ⅓ cup skim milk
1 handful of parsley leaves, chopped
sea salt and ground white pepper

1 Put a large saucepan over medium heat and spray with oil. Fry the onion for 3–4 minutes until soft, then add the garlic and cook for 1 minute.
2 Add the remaining ingredients, except the parsley and seasoning. Bring to a boil, then reduce the heat to a simmer and cook for 20–25 minutes until the beans are tender. Add the parsley, season with salt and pepper, and serve.

Nutritional information per serving
Kcals **340** Protein **33g** Carbohydrate **49g** Fat **3g**

Best for Stress Hunger. Stress burns up B vitamins, which help us to release energy from food. This is one reason you feel so tired (and often pig out on sugary treats) when stressed. Beans are a great source of B vitamins, which help to boost energy and reduce stress overeating. Also good for

Edamame and Basil Soup

Many of us have eaten edamame beans in Japanese restaurants without realizing these are actually soybeans. The good thing about them is that they have the highest protein content of the bean family as well as being delicious. You can buy them fresh in some supermarkets now, or you can buy frozen ones from Asian suppliers and in many other markets.

Serves: 4
Preparation time: 10 minutes
Cooking time: 15 minutes, plus cooling

1½ cups fresh podded edamame beans

1½ cups frozen peas
4 cups vegetable bouillon
6 scallions, chopped
1 large bunch basil, leaves chopped
1 bunch arugula
generous ¾ cup skim milk

1 Put the edamame beans, peas and bouillon in a large saucepan, bring to a boil and simmer for 5 minutes. Add the remaining ingredients and cook for another 5 minutes.

2 Remove from the heat to cool slightly. Transfer half the mixture to a blender or food processor and blend until smooth. Pour it back into the pan with the chunky mixture, return to the heat and bring back to a boil, then serve.

Nutritional information per serving
Kcals **240** Protein **11g** Carbohydrate **11g** Fat **3g**

Best for Anxious Hunger. Edamame—aka soybeans—have the highest protein of all the beans, so are great for keeping your blood sugar level. This can prevent cravings and overeating, for Anxious Types and many others. Also good for

Tuscan Tomato Soup

Canned cream of tomato soup is, I think, the most hideous soup ever invented—gloopy and metallic tasting—and yet tomatoes themselves make a great soup base. This recipe is full of flavor. It's hearty but low in calories.

Serves: 4
Preparation time: 15 minutes
Cooking time: 40 minutes, plus cooling

olive oil spray
1 small red onion, finely chopped
1 garlic clove, crushed
1 carrot, peeled and chopped

2 celery stalks, chopped
scant 3½ cups vegetable bouillon
1 x 14oz can chopped tomatoes
1 x 14oz can mixed beans, drained and rinsed
1 tablespoon tomato paste
leaves of 2 thyme sprigs
sea salt and freshly ground black pepper

1 Put a large nonstick saucepan over medium heat and spray with oil. Fry the onion for 3–4 minutes until soft. Add the garlic, carrot and celery, and cook for 5 minutes (add a little of the bouillon if the mixture sticks to the pan).
2 Add the remaining ingredients and bring to a boil, then reduce the heat, cover and simmer for 20–30 minutes until the vegetables are cooked. Remove from the heat and leave to cool slightly.
3 Transfer half the mixture to a blender or food processor and blend until smooth. Pour it back into the pan with the chunky mixture, return to the heat and bring back to a boil, then serve.

Nutritional information per serving
Kcals **172** Protein **8g** Carbohydrate **22g** Fat **5g**

 Best for Stress Hunger. Celery contains compounds called phthalides, which relax the blood vessels, thus reducing blood pressure. This is helpful for weight loss because stress and anxiety are common overeating triggers. Being relaxed may help you make better food choices. Also good for 🥣 🥣 🥣 🥣 🥣

Moroccan Fava Bean Soup

Here's another twist on boring old vegetable soup. This one has Moroccan flavors and is lovely and silky, due to the fava beans.

Serves: 4
Preparation time: 15 minutes
Cooking time: 20 minutes

olive oil spray
1 onion, chopped
2 celery stalks, chopped
1 garlic clove, crushed
2 teaspoons ground cumin

1 teaspoon harissa paste
4 cups vegetable bouillon
1 x 14oz can chopped tomatoes
2⅔ cups frozen fava or lima beans
zest and juice of 1 lemon
1 large handful each of cilantro and
    parsley leaves, chopped
sea salt and freshly ground black
    pepper

1 Put a nonstick saucepan over medium heat and spray with oil, then fry the onion and celery for 3–4 minutes. Add the garlic, cumin and harissa, and fry for 1 minute (add a splash of water if the mixture sticks to the pan).
2 Add the bouillon, tomatoes and fava beans, then bring to a boil. Reduce the heat, cover and simmer for 10 minutes. Add the lemon zest and juice, then season with salt and pepper. Remove the pan from the heat.
3 Transfer half the mixture to a blender or food processor and blend until smooth. Pour it back into the pan with the chunky mixture, return to the heat and bring back to a boil. Stir in the herbs and serve.

Nutritional information per serving
Kcals **116** Protein **31g** Carbohydrate **64g** Fat **4g**

Best for Tired Hunger. Herbs and spices are not just great tasting, they also have some of the highest concentrations of important nutrients of any vegetables. Cumin is full of iron, which boosts energy and can help tired overeaters. Also good for 🥣 🥣 🥣 🥣

Spicy Lentil Soup

There are loads of ways to make lentil soup, but I like it spiced. The lemon halves are important to give a subtle, but definite, citrus tang.

Serves: 4
Preparation time: 10 minutes
Cooking time: 40 minutes, plus cooling

olive oil spray
1 onion, chopped
1 garlic clove, chopped
1 teaspoon ground ginger
1 teaspoon garam masala

4 cups vegetable bouillon
1 carrot, peeled and chopped
1 parsnip, peeled and chopped
1 lemon, cut in half
¾ cup dried Puy lentils
sea salt and freshly ground black pepper
4 tablespoons fat-free Greek yogurt, to serve

1 Put a large nonstick saucepan over medium heat and spray with oil, then fry the onion for 3–4 minutes to soften. Add the garlic and cook for 1 minute, then add the spices and cook for 1 minute.

2 Pour in the bouillon, vegetables, lemon and lentils. Bring to a boil, then reduce the heat, cover and simmer for 25–30 minutes until the lentils are soft. Remove the pan from the heat and leave to cool slightly. Remove the lemon. Transfer to a blender or food processor and blend until smooth. Season with salt and pepper, then stir in the yogurt and serve.

Nutritional information per serving
Kcals **255** Protein **11g** Carbohydrate **30g** Fat **5g**

Best for Anxious Hunger. There's a reason veggies are so chilled out. Lentils contain glutamic acid, which the body converts into the anti-anxiety neurotransmitter GABA. This can reduce anxious and stress eating. Also good for

Mexican Pinto Bean Soup with Avocado Salsa

....

Pinto beans are those slightly mottled beans you sometimes see dried, but it's probably more convenient to use canned kidney beans. Either way, don't skip the avocado salsa. The cool and silky salsa with the hot, chunky soup is a real winner.

Serves: 4
Preparation time: 15 minutes
Cooking time: 1 hour

olive oil spray
1 onion, chopped
6 garlic cloves, crushed
1 red chili, seeded and chopped
1 teaspoon cayenne pepper
1 teaspoon ground cumin
1 teaspoon ground coriander
1 teaspoon smoked paprika
1 red bell pepper, seeded and
   roughly chopped
1 yellow bell pepper, seeded and roughly chopped
2 tablespoons red wine vinegar
1 tablespoons stevia-based granulated sweetener
2 tablespoons tomato paste
1 x 14oz can pinto or red kidney beans, drained and rinsed
2 x 14oz cans chopped tomatoes
generous 1½ cups vegetable bouillon
sea salt and freshly ground black pepper

For the avocado salsa
1 ripe avocado, peeled, pitted and diced
½ red onion, finely sliced
½ red chili, seeded and finely sliced
1 tablespoon chopped cilantro leaves
juice of 1 lime
1 tablespoon olive oil
a pinch of sea salt

1 Put a large nonstick saucepan over medium heat and spray with oil, then fry the onion for 3–4 minutes until soft. Add the garlic, chili, spices and bell peppers, and cook for 5 minutes (add a splash of water if the mixture sticks to the pan).

2 Add the vinegar, sweetener and tomato paste, and cook for 5 minutes. Add the beans, tomatoes and bouillon. Season with salt and pepper, and bring to a boil, then reduce the heat, cover and simmer for 40 minutes.

3 To make the avocado salsa, mix all the ingredients together. Serve the soup with a dollop of the salsa on top.

Nutritional information per serving
Kcals **281** Protein **11g** Carbohydrate **33g** Fat **14g**

 Best for Never-Full Hunger. Unbalanced blood sugar can cause mood swings and sugar cravings. The compound that gives the heat to chilies, capsaicin, helps to balance blood sugar. Also good for

Miso Soup with Butternut Squash and Tofu

Traditional Japanese miso soup is made from a bouillon containing fermented soya beans. This may not sound very appetizing, but it gives the bouillon, called dashi, a fantastic tangy flavor. I've included a recipe for that here, or you can cheat and buy dashi bouillon in health food shops.

Serves: 4
Preparation time: 15 minutes, plus 1 hour soaking
Cooking time: 25 minutes, plus standing

1lb butternut squash, with skin, seeded and cut into chunks
8oz snow peas

4 tablespoons miso
15oz firm tofu, drained, rinsed and cubed

For the dashi
1 x 5-inch strip of dried kombu (Japanese seaweed)
2 tablespoons dried bonito flakes

1 To make the dashi, soak the kombu in a saucepan with 5¼ cups water for 1 hour. Bring the water to a boil, but remove the kombu just before the water reaches boiling point. Add the bonito flakes and simmer gently for 5 minutes. Remove from the heat and leave to stand for 5 minutes, then strain the liquid through a sieve into a large pitcher.

2 Put the squash in a steamer over a pan of boiling water and steam for 15 minutes until tender. Turn off the heat and leave to cool. Steam the snow peas for 2 minutes or until still a little crunchy. Transfer to a colander and refresh under cold water. Drain and set aside. Scoop out the squash flesh from the peel and put it into a blender or food processor, then blend until smooth. Add the miso and mix well. Heat the dashi in a saucepan over medium heat and gradually stir in the squash, then bring the mixture up to a gentle simmer. Add the tofu and snow peas, heat through and serve.

Nutritional information per serving
Kcals **123** Protein **25g** Carbohydrate **3g** Fat **5g**

Best for PMS Hunger. Miso is a source of plant estrogens called phytestrogens. These have been shown to improve PMS, a common trigger for overeating, and post menopausal weight gain. Also good for

SANDWICHES

Who doesn't love a sandwich at lunchtime? Quick, convenient and the perfect at-your-desk meal. The problem with store-bought sandwiches, though, is both the quality of the bread and that there's too much of it. It turns what could be a balanced meal into a carb attack, which unbalances blood sugar and leads to mid-afternoon tiredness and the inevitable cookie munchies.

I've come up with some ideas for Hunger Type sandwiches. These all increase protein, healthy fats and fiber, to slow down the post-sandwich blood sugar rise while keeping calories under control. I have included some home-baked bread options. If you don't want to go that far, try to buy bread that has been made properly. Avoid mass-produced white, brown and malted breads that feel soft. Look out for rye, spelt, millet, buckwheat or sourdough—the traditional grains and their slower fermentation process makes them healthier.

Sandwich fillings

A sandwich doesn't have to be two slices of bread with something sad in between. Great sandwiches are made of great bread combined with interesting fillings, strong flavors and plenty of texture from nuts, vegetables or crisp salad leaves.

All of the fillings here work best when you also add a handful of mixed leaves, because they bulk up the sandwich for very few calories and increase the nutrient content. Plus, leaves "insulate" the bread from the filling, stopping it from going soggy, which is especially important if you're making them in the morning and not eating them until lunchtime.

Spelt and Seed Loaf

Although a type of wheat, spelt is a more traditional form and has a lower GI than modern wheat. This means it releases its energy more slowly into your body, thereby preventing a spike and then a cravings-triggering slump later on.

Makes: 1 loaf (10 slices)
Preparation time: 20 minutes, plus 2¾ hours rising
Baking time: 35 minutes, plus cooling

2¼ teaspoons active dry yeast
2 tablespoons agave syrup

heaping 3¾ cups spelt flour, plus extra for dusting
2 teaspoons sea salt
2 tablespoons sunflower seeds
2 tablespoons sesame seeds
olive oil spray

1 Put the yeast in a small bowl and add 1¼ cups warm water and the agave syrup. Leave for 10 minutes until frothy.
2 In another bowl, mix the flour, salt and seeds together, then make a well in the center and pour in the yeast mixture. Use your hands to combine the ingredients into a smooth, non-sticky dough.
3 Lightly flour the work surface. Knead the dough for 5 minutes, then put it back in the bowl and cover with plastic wrap. Leave in a warm place for 1 hour or until it has doubled in size.
4 Turn the dough out onto a floured work surface, knead for 3 minutes, then put back in the bowl, cover with plastic wrap and leave to rise again for 1½ hours.
5 Preheat the oven to 375°F and spray a baking sheet with olive oil spray. Turn the dough out of the bowl onto the prepared baking sheet. Slash the top of the loaf with a sharp knife and Bake for 30–35 minutes until it sounds hollow when tapped underneath. Leave on a wire rack to cool completely. Cut into 10 slices to serve.

Nutritional information per slice
Kcals **154** Protein **5g** Carbohydrate **4g** Fat **1g**

Best for Stress Hunger. Sesame and sunflower seeds contain tryptophan, which is converted into serotonin to suppress the appetite. Fats from the seeds are helpful to combat stress. Also good for

No-Knead Buckwheat Bread

Buckwheat is actually a seed, not a grain, so it's gluten-free (which is why it doesn't need kneading) and is high in Hunger Type-friendly omega-3 fats. It is dense calorifically, though, so you will need to slice this one thinly.

Makes: 1 loaf (15 slices)
Preparation time: 15 minutes, plus 1¼ hours rising
Baking time: 30 minutes, plus cooling

olive oil spray
2¼ teaspoons active dry yeast
2 teaspoons stevia-based granulated sweetener

2 eggs
2 tablespoons olive oil
5 cups buckwheat flour or 3⅓ cups buckwheat groats ground to a powder in a food processor
1 teaspoon sea salt
1 teaspoon vinegar

1 Spray an 8 x 4 x 2-inch loaf pan with oil. Put the yeast and sweetener in a small bowl and add a scant 1½ cups warm water. Leave for 10 minutes until frothy.

2 In another bowl, beat the eggs and oil together until frothy. Put the flour and salt in another bowl, make a well in the center and add the egg mixture, vinegar and the yeast mixture. Stir together until you have a wet mixture that is more like a very thick batter than a dough.

3 Pour the batter into the prepared loaf pan and cover with oiled plastic wrap. Leave in a warm place for 30 minutes–1 hour to rise—you want a lift, but if you let it rise too much it will collapse in the oven.

4 Preheat the oven to 375°F. Remove the plastic wrap and bake the bread for 25–30 minutes until a toothpick inserted into the center comes out clean.

Leave on a wire rack to cool completely. Cut into 15 slices to serve.

Nutritional information per slice
Kcals **149** Protein **6g** Carbohydrate **23g** Fat **3g**

Best for Tired Hunger. Tiredness can stop dieters exercising and make them reach for the nearest convenient, high-cal snack. Buckwheat contains energy-boosting B vitamins and iron to stop this. Also good for

Chickpea and Rosemary Bread

Adding herbs to bread (and other foods) isn't just about giving them great flavor. Herbs are higher in important nutrients than most fruits and vegetables. The rosemary in this bread has been shown to boost memory. It tastes lovely too.

Makes: 1 loaf (15 slices)
Preparation time: 25 minutes, plus 2 hours rising
Baking time: 30 minutes, plus cooling

1 x 14oz can chickpeas, drained and rinsed

Heaping 3¾ cups whole-wheat flour, plus extra for dusting
2¼ teaspoons active dry yeast
1 tablespoon chopped rosemary leaves or 1 teaspoon dried rosemary
zest and juice of ½ lemon
olive oil spray

1 Make sure the rinsed chickpeas are well-drained in a colander, then remove the skins and put the chickpeas in a food processor. Process them to a rough crumb. Pour into a large bowl and add the flour, yeast, rosemary, and lemon zest and juice. Stir together using a wooden spoon.

2 Gradually add about 1 cup warm water until you get a soft dough. Turn out onto a floured work surface and knead for 10 minutes. Put back in the bowl, cover with oiled plastic wrap and leave in a warm place for 2 hours or until the dough has doubled in size.

3 Preheat the oven to 425°F and spray an 8 x 4 x 2-inch loaf pan with oil. Remove the dough from the bowl and knead again for 1 minute. Put into the prepared pan and bake for 30 minutes or until a toothpick inserted into the center comes out clean. Leave on a wire rack to cool completely. Cut into 15 thin slices to serve.

Nutritional information per slice
Kcals **138** Protein **6g** Carbohydrate **6g** Fat **1g**

Best for 40+ Hunger. Chickpeas don't just fill you up with fiber, they are also a helpful diet food. The phytoestrogens they contain can lower estrogen levels, which promote fat storage, in both men and women. Also good for 🍵 🌙 ❄️

Whole-Wheat Pita Breads

Pita breads are great because they are portion controlled. Plus, they make a fantastic portable lunch.

Makes: 6 pita breads
Preparation time: 25 minutes, plus 2 hours rising
Baking time: 20 minutes, plus cooling

Heaping 3¾ cups whole-wheat flour, plus extra for dusting
2¼ teaspoons active dry yeast
1 teaspoon sea salt
1 tablespoon olive oil
olive oil spray

1 Put the flour, yeast and salt in a large bowl. Add the oil and gradually add about a scant 1¼ cups warm water until you get a soft dough. Turn out onto a floured work surface and knead for 5–10 minutes until soft and stretchy.
2 Put back in the bowl, cover with oiled plastic wrap and leave in a warm place for 1–2 hours or until the dough has doubled in size.
3 Preheat the oven to 500°F and put a baking sheet in the oven to heat up. Turn out the dough and knead for 1 minute. Divide it into 6 equal balls and flatten them to ¼-inch thick.
4 Using oven gloves, remove the baking sheet from the oven, dust with flour and put the dough discs on it, leaving space between each one. You will probably have to bake the dough in two batches. Bake for 5–10 minutes until they have puffed up and are lightly golden. Leave on a wire rack to cool completely. Split the pita breads and fill to serve.

Nutritional information per pita bread
Kcals **290** Protein **10g** Carbohydrate **5g** Fat **4g**

Best for Stress Hunger. Pita breads have a lower GI than many "normal" sliced breads. This means they can help keep blood sugar and hunger hormones stable—essential for Stress Hunger, particularly. Also good for

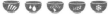

Brown Rice Wraps

These wraps are really quick to make. There's no kneading and no "leaving to rise" time. You simply make a batter and pour it into a pan. Plus, if you pour the batter thinly, they are less "bready", so the carb load is reduced and you can have more filling and less sandwich. You can substitute whole-wheat flour, if you can't get brown rice flour.

Makes: 6 wraps
Preparation time: 25 minutes, plus 25 minutes standing
Baking time: 15 minutes

1½ cups brown rice flour
4 teaspoons olive oil
a pinch of sea salt
olive oil spray

1 Put the flour, olive oil and salt in a large bowl and add a scant 1⅓ cups water, then stir together using a wooden spoon to form a smooth batter. Leave to stand for 20–25 minutes.
2 Put a nonstick skillet over medium heat and spray with oil. Pour in 2–3 tablespoons of the batter and smooth it out to form a pancake. Cook until bubbles form on the surface, then flip the pancake over to cook the other side. Turn out onto a plate and repeat with the remaining batter. Serve with a filling (see pages 257–263).

Nutritional information per wrap
Kcals **159** Protein **2g** Carbohydrate **2g** Fat **4g**

 Best for Anxious Hunger. Rice bran contains glutamic acid, which the body uses to make anxiety-reducing GABA, thus helping to reduce anxious comfort eating. Also good for

Marrakesh Chicken Salad

This is a filling with a balance of sweet and savory. It works really well inside a pita bread, as it tends to fall out of a sandwich.

Serves: 2
Preparation time: 15 minutes

4 tablespoons fat-free Greek yogurt
1 teaspoon agave syrup
a squeeze of lemon juice
a pinch of sea salt
a pinch of ground cumin

a pinch of ground cinnamon
a pinch of cayenne pepper
scant ¾ cup shredded cooked
    skinless chicken breast
1 carrot, peeled and grated
1 pitted dried date, chopped
2 Whole-Wheat Pita Breads (see page
    255), to serve

1 Put the yogurt in a bowl and add the agave syrup, lemon juice, salt and spices. Stir well to combine, then stir in the chicken, carrot and date.
2 Slice the pita breads through the edges to form pockets and fill with the chicken mixture. Serve.

Nutritional information per serving of filling (in addition to the pitta)
Kcals **153** Protein **18g** Carbohydrate **16g** Fat **2g**

Best for Winter-Blues Hunger. Dates are both high in the amino acid tryptophan, which we need to make the natural antidepressant and the appetite-suppressant hormone serotonin, and they also contain sugar, which potentiates its effect. Also good for

Turkey Cranberry

Cranberries and turkey are a traditional pairing. Rather than sugary cranberry sauce, though, I've used dried cranberries here for natural sweetness.

Serves: 2
Preparation time: 10 minutes

⅔ cup cooked chopped turkey breast
1 tablespoon dried cranberries
2 tablespoons fat-free Greek yogurt
¼ red onion, finely chopped
1 handful of lamb's lettuce
4 slices of bread, to serve

1 Put all the ingredients, except the lamb's lettuce, in a bowl and mix them together well.
2 Put some lamb's lettuce on top of two slices of bread. Divide the filling between them and top with more lettuce and another slice of bread. Serve.

Nutritional information per serving of filling (in addition to the bread)
Kcals **112** Protein **17g** Carbohydrate **6g** Fat **2g**

Best for Never-Full Hunger. Cranberries are not only bursting with healthy phytonutrients but they are also high in soluble fiber. This swells up in your gut, improving digestion and helping you feel full. Also good for

Tuna with a Kick

I once went on a vacation and we had so little money that I packed cans of tuna in my suitcase so that I could make tuna mayonnaise sandwiches for lunch. It was a cheap, but not very slimming, vacation diet. My Hunger Type tuna mayo is much better for you.

Serves: 2
Preparation time: 10 minutes, plus chiling

¼ cup very low-fat cottage cheese
½ teaspoon dried chili flakes
5oz canned tuna in spring water, drained

a squeeze of lemon juice
1 celery stalk, chopped
1 bunch of watercress
sea salt and freshly ground black pepper
4 slices of bread, to serve

1 Put the cottage cheese into a blender or food processor and add the chili flakes, tuna and lemon juice. Blend until smooth, then pour into a bowl and add the celery. Season with salt and pepper. Chill in the fridge to firm up before using.
2 Put some watercress on two slices of bread. Divide the filling between them and top with more watercress and another slice of bread. Serve.

Nutritional information per serving of filling (in addition to the bread)
Kcals **98** Protein **20g** Carbohydrate **trace** Fat **trace**

Best for Hedonistic Hunger. Celery is what is known as a negative calorie food (NCF). The NCF theory is that it takes more calories to digest celery than it contains, so you actually burn calories by eating it. Also good for

Updated Shrimp Cocktail

Shrimp cocktail was that awful sticky-sweet 1980s' steak-house starter, and anyone who remembers differently is allowing nostalgia to cloud their judgement. Still, the combination of shrimp and avocado is a good one. It just needs lightening up.

Serves: 2
Preparation time: 15 minutes

1 tablespoon extra-virgin olive oil
1 teaspoon lemon juice
3½oz cooked, peeled shrimp
½ fennel bulb, very thinly sliced

1 handful of arugula
½ avocado, cut in half, pitted, peeled and thinly sliced
2 scallions, chopped
sea salt and freshly ground black pepper
4 slices of bread, to serve

1 Put the oil in a bowl and add the lemon juice. Season to taste with salt and pepper, then mix well together. Add the shrimp and fennel, and gently coat with the oil mixture.
2 Put some arugula on two slices of bread and divide the filling between them. Top with the avocado and sprinkle with the scallions. Top with more arugula and another slice of bread. Serve.

Nutritional information per serving of filling (in addition to the bread)
Kcals **115** Protein **8g** Carbohydrate **4g** Fat **6g**

Best for Never-Full Hunger. The hormone leptin requires zinc—contained in shrimp—to work properly and switch off hunger. Also good for 🥣 🥣 🥣

Thai-Style Crayfish and Cucumber

Shrimp and cucumber can be a real yawn. This recipe uses crayfish, which are a pest to our native river life so we need to eat more of them—and they give the filling an interesting twist.

Serves: 2
Preparation time: 5 minutes

4 tablespoons fat-free Greek yogurt
¼ teaspoon Thai curry paste
5½oz cooked, peeled crayfish or shrimp

½ cucumber, sliced
a squeeze of lemon juice
1 tablespoon chopped cilantro leaves
8 butterhead lettuce leaves
4 slices of bread, to serve

1 Put the yogurt in a bowl and stir in the curry paste. Add the crayfish, cucumber, lemon juice and cilantro, and gently combine.
2 Put 2 lettuce leaves on two slices of bread and divide the filling between them. Top with two more lettuce leaves and a slice of bread each. Serve.

Nutritional information per serving of filling (in addition to the bread)
Kcals **85** Protein **15g** Carbohydrate **3g** Fat **1g**

 Best for Stress Hunger. Cilantro leaf has a high concentration of important nutrients, including B vitamins, which help the body deal with stress and so may reduce stress eating. Also good for

Spiced Egg Salad

Any chance to include eggs in your diet is a good one. This is a meat-free version of Coronation Chicken.

Serves: 2
Preparation time: 10 minutes
Cooking time: 10 minutes, plus cooling

1 egg
2 tablespoons fat-free Greek yogurt
½ teaspoon curry powder
a pinch of sea salt
½ red bell pepper, seeded and chopped
4 lettuce leaves
4 slices of bread, to serve

1 Put the egg in a pan of boiling water and cook for 10 minutes. Drain the egg and put it into a bowl of cold water to cool. Peel off the shell, then chop the egg.

2 Put the yogurt in a bowl and add the curry powder and salt. Stir to combine, then add the bell pepper and egg, and stir gently to coat. Put a lettuce leaf on two slices of bread. Divide the egg mixture between the two, then top with another lettuce leaf and another slice of bread. Serve.

Nutritional information per serving of filling (in addition to the bread)
Kcals **78** Protein **3g** Carbohydrate **2g** Fat **7g**

 Best for Tired Hunger. Low levels of the sleep hormone melatonin can cause insomnia and increased appetite. Bell peppers, however, are high in vitamin C, which is used to make melatonin, so they can help with sleep.
Also good for

Cottage Cheese and Walnut Slaw

"Normal" coleslaw is incredibly fattening. This one has added protein from the cottage cheese and a much lower calorie dressing.

Serves: 2
Preparation time: 10 minutes

1 carrot, peeled and grated
⅓ cup fresh beansprouts
¼ red onion, chopped

heaping ⅓ cup very low-fat cottage
    cheese
1½ tablespoons chopped walnuts
1 teaspoon sesame seeds
1 handful of baby spinach leaves
4 slices of bread, to serve

1 Put all the ingredients, except the spinach, in a large bowl and mix together.
2 Put half the spinach on two slices of bread and add the filling, then cover with the remaining spinach and the other slices of bread. Serve.

Nutritional information per serving of filling (in addition to the bread)
Kcals **83** Protein **8g** Carbohydrate **6g** Fat **5g**

Best for Cravings Hunger. Cottage cheese is a good source of tyrosine, which converts to the anti-craving neurotransmitter dopamine in the body. Also good for 🥣 🥣 🥣 🥣

LUNCH POTS

Some nutritionists and food snobs look down on the microwave. And, yes, it probably is less healthy than cooking your food over cedar chips while breathing in fresh mountain air. But let's get real—how many people have the time to cook lunch from scratch? Sometimes the microwave is the only way.

As a reflection of this, we can see the popularity of the microwaveable lunch pot. Some of them are pretty nutritionally hair-raising (white rice with a glob of MSG-laden sweet-'n'-sour sauce anyone?), but they don't have to be. It's pretty easy to make your own version at home and, because they are eaten hot, they feel substantial. If a salad or a soup doesn't feel enough for you for lunch, try one of these.

Sweet-and-Sour Pork Lunch Pot

This is my version of the famous takeout. I've left out the pineapple, because its GI is too high, but I also think it's too sweet with that anyway.

Serves: 2
Preparation time: 15 minutes
Cooking time: 50 minutes, plus cooling

¾ cup uncooked brown rice (or 1½ cups cooked rice—see method for cooling)
1 tablespoon cornstarch
1 teaspoon soy sauce

1 tablespoon tomato paste
1 teaspoon stevia-based granulated sweetener
3 tablespoons rice wine vinegar
olive oil spray
7oz lean pork, cut into small pieces
½ red bell pepper, seeded and chopped
½ green bell pepper, seeded and chopped

1 If you are using uncooked rice, put it in a large saucepan and cover generously with water. Bring to a boil, then simmer for 35–40 minutes until tender. Drain in a sieve, then transfer the rice onto a large plate, spread it out and leave it to cool. As soon as it is cold, put it in the fridge until needed.
2 Put the cornstarch in a small bowl and add a scant ¼ cup water. Stir until smooth. Add the soy sauce, tomato paste, sweetener and vinegar, and stir to combine. Put a wok or large saucepan over medium-high heat and spray with oil, then stir-fry the pork for 2–3 minutes. Remove the pork and set aside. Add the bell peppers and stir-fry for 2–3 minutes (add a splash of water if the mixture sticks to the pan).
3 Pour in the cornstarch mixture and cook for 2–3 minutes, stirring, then put the pork back into the wok and stir for 1 minute. Leave to cool completely. Put the rice into plastic lunch-sized pots and top with the pork mixture. Seal the pots ready for taking with you. Chill until using. Reheat in a microwave at full power for 3½ minutes.

Nutritional information per serving
Kcals **342** Protein **28g** Carbohydrate **44g** Fat **6g**

 Best for 40+ Hunger. The thyroid controls metabolic rate and requires selenium, found in pork. As the thyroid can decline with age, selenium may benefit it. Also good for

Provençale Tuna and Ratatouille Lunch Pot

Ratatouille is a useful diet staple, with added protein. You could make a big batch and use some for soup, some as a lunch pot and some as a cold salsa.

Serves: 2
Preparation time:
Cooking time: 1 hour 10 minutes, plus cooling

½ cup uncooked brown rice (or 1 cup cooked brown rice)
olive oil spray
½ onion, chopped
1 red bell pepper, seeded and chopped
1 garlic clove, crushed
1 rosemary sprig
½ eggplant, diced
1 zucchini, diced
1 x 14oz can chopped tomatoes
1 teaspoon balsamic vinegar
6oz canned tuna steak in spring water, drained and flaked
1 handful of basil leaves, shredded

1 If you are using uncooked rice, put it in a large saucepan and cover generously with water. Bring to the boil and simmer for 35–40 minutes until tender. Drain in a sieve, then transfer the rice onto a large plate, spread it out and leave it to cool. As soon as it is cold, put it in the fridge until needed.
2 Put a nonstick saucepan over medium heat and spray with oil, then fry the onion and bell pepper for 5 minutes or until soft. Add the garlic and cook for another 1 minute (add a splash of water if the mixture sticks to the pan).
3 Add the rosemary, eggplant, zucchini and tomatoes. Bring to a boil, then reduce the heat and simmer, uncovered, for 20 minutes or until the vegetables are cooked and the sauce has reduced. Stir in the vinegar, then leave to cool.
4 Put the rice in plastic lunch-sized pots followed by the ratatouille, and top each with half the tuna and the basil. Seal the pots ready for taking with you. Chill until using. Reheat in a microwave at full power for 3½ minutes.

Nutritional information per serving
Kcals **292** Protein **39g** Carbohydrate **35g** Fat **5g**

Best for Emotional Hunger, because the tomatoes in ratatouille are high in natural sugars that can help boost serotonin. Also good for

Shrimp, Quinoa and Paprika Paella Lunch Pot

My oil-free paella uses cauliflower instead of rice and is healthy and tasty.

Serves: 2
Preparation time: 15 minutes
Cooking time: 25 minutes, plus cooling

7oz raw large shrimp, peeled
2 garlic cloves, crushed
zest and juice of ½ lemon
1 teaspoon smoked paprika

a pinch of sea salt
olive oil spray
1 onion, chopped
scant ⅔ cup quinoa
1 teaspoon ground turmeric
4 cups roughly chopped cauliflower florets
⅓ cup frozen peas
1 tablespoon chopped parsley leaves

1 Devein the shrimp as described in step 1 on page 242. Set aside. Put the garlic in a bowl and add the lemon juice and zest, paprika and salt. Mix well to combine, then add the shrimp, stirring to coat them in the mixture. Set aside.

2 Put a nonstick saucepan over medium heat and spray with oil, then fry the onion for 5 minutes until soft. Add the quinoa, turmeric and a generous 1½ cups water. Bring to a boil, then reduce the heat, cover and simmer for 10 minutes or until almost tender.

3 Meanwhile, put the cauliflower into a food processor and process until the consistency of rice. Add to the quinoa, followed by the peas, then bring back to a boil and cover. Simmer for 5 minutes or until the quinoa is tender and the peas are cooked. Remove the pan from the heat.

4 Put a nonstick skillet over medium heat and spray with oil, then fry the shrimp for 1–2 minutes on each side until pink. Leave everything to cool, then put the quinoa into plastic lunch-sized pots, add the shrimp and sprinkle with parsley. Seal the pots ready for taking with you. Chill until using. Reheat in a microwave at full power for 3½ minutes.

Nutritional information per serving
Kcals **395** Protein **77g** Carbohydrate **52g** Fat **12g**

Best for Never-Full Hunger. Paprika, from the chili family, is thermogenic. It could speed up metabolism, helping you burn more calories. Also good for

Eastern Chickpea, Coconut and Spinach Lunch Pot

This is a lighter version of a Thai vegetable curry with spinach instead of rice.

Serves: 2
Preparation time: 15 minutes
Cooking time: 25 minutes, plus cooling

10½oz baby spinach leaves
olive oil spray
½ small onion, chopped
2 garlic cloves, crushed
1-inch piece of ginger root, grated
1 tablespoon tomato paste
zest and juice of ½ lemon
a pinch of dried chili flakes
1 x 14oz can chickpeas, drained and rinsed
generous ¾ cup reduced-fat coconut milk
a pinch of ground ginger
½ teaspoon stevia-based granulated sweetener

1 Thinly slice a few of the spinach leaves and set aside. Put a nonstick saucepan over medium heat and spray with oil, then fry the onion for 5 minutes or until soft. Add the garlic, grated ginger, tomato paste, lemon zest and chili flakes, and fry for 3 minutes, stirring (add some water if the mixture sticks to the pan).

2 Add the chickpeas and cook for 3 minutes, stirring to coat them in the mixture, then gradually add the remaining unsliced spinach, pressing it down and turning it over using tongs as it begins to wilt. Pour in the coconut milk, ground ginger and sweetener, then simmer gently for 10 minutes.

3 Stir in the lemon juice and leave to cool. Pour the mixture into plastic lunch-sized pots and top with the reserved spinach. Seal the pots ready for taking with you. Chill until using. Reheat in a microwave at full power for 3½ minutes.

Nutritional information per serving
Kcals **342** Protein **15g** Carbohydrate **38g** Fat **11g**

Best for 40+ Hunger. Coconut has been shown to improve thyroid function. The thyroid is the gland that controls your metabolic rate (how fast you burn calories), and a healthy thyroid helps you lose weight. Also good for 🥣 🥣 🥣 🥣

Dhal with Broccoli Lunch Pot

Spicy dhal is a perfect dish to put in a lunch pot. It doesn't dry out, it travels well and it can be easily revived in a microwave. I haven't added any rice, quinoa or other grain to this, as lentils not only contain protein but are also already quite high in carbs. They make a balanced meal in themselves.

Serves: 2
Preparation time: 15 minutes
Cooking time: 30 minutes, plus cooling

scant ⅔ cup red lentils
1 teaspoon ground turmeric
1 tablespoon tamarind paste
a pinch of sea salt

olive oil spray
1 onion, finely chopped
1 garlic clove, crushed
1¼-inch piece of ginger root, peeled and grated
1 teaspoon curry powder
9oz broccoli, broken into small florets, stem discarded

1 Put the lentils in a medium saucepan over medium heat and add ½ cup water, the turmeric, tamarind and salt. Bring to a boil, then cover and simmer for 15 minutes or until the lentils are soft.
2 Meanwhile, put a nonstick skillet over medium heat and spray with oil, then fry the onion for 5 minutes or until soft. Add the garlic and ginger, and cook for 2 minutes (add a splash of water if the mixture sticks to the pan). Stir in the curry powder and cook for 2 minutes.
3 Pour in the lentils and cook for 10 minutes, then leave to cool. Meanwhile, put the broccoli in a steamer over a pan of boiling water and steam for 5 minutes or until tender. Transfer to a colander and refresh under cold water. Drain and set aside to cool. Pour the dhal into plastic lunch-sized pots and top with the broccoli. Seal the pots ready for taking with you. Chill until using. Reheat in a microwave at full power for 3½ minutes.

Nutritional information per serving
Kcals **335** Protein **24g** Carbohydrate **50g** Fat **26g**

Best for Anxious Hunger. Lentils can reduce anxious overeating, because they are a good source of glutamic acid, which our bodies convert into the anti-anxiety hormone GABA. Also good for

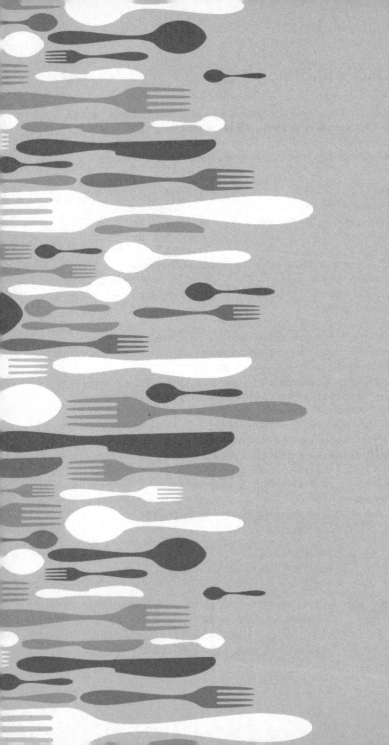

Snacks

The idea of eating little and often is great—in theory—but for many, if you are a Hunger Type, this can turn into eating too much and constantly. In my experience while helping people lose weight, those who lose most are the ones who stick to a regular eating pattern of three meals a day; however, that gap between lunch and dinner can seem like a yawning chasm, one that is too easily filled with trips to a convenience store, office vending machine or home fridge. With this in mind, I have designed some Hunger Type snacks. If you can do without them, you will lose weight faster, but if you know that minus an afternoon snack you will arrive home like a hungry pterodactyl and eat everything in sight, then add one snack between three and five o'clock.

SAVORY SNACKS

Raw veg and dips

This is my favorite snack for my weight-loss clients. The combination of crunchy raw veg and smooth dip is a good one, because the veg provides something to chew for very few calories. The act of chewing is like a stress ball for some, particularly Anxious Hunger Types.

Just remember that this is a snack, not a meal, so don't go mad. The portion size of vegetables should be no more than can sit in the palm of your hand. Choose from carrot sticks, cucumber sticks, snow peas, baby corn, sugar snap peas, scallions or a couple of asparagus spears or celery stalks.

The obvious dip is hummus, but this can be very high in fat and a bit heavy on the carbs. I've started instead with a recipe for a lighter version. Like the other dips here, it has added protein in the form of yogurt to stabilize energy and mood.

Filled eggs

Yes, I know, eggs again! But they are a fantastically nutritious food and great for weight loss. I'm not suggesting you eat a half-dozen a day, but if you haven't had them as part of one of your meals, then boiled eggs make a good snack, especially if filled. All of these can be made a day in advance and stored in the fridge, although you'll need to wrap the Guacamole Eggs in plastic wrap to stop them turning brown.

Smoked Salmon and Dill Dip

Smoked salmon dips are usually made with cream, but they work just as well with yogurt, plus it adds a pleasant tartness.

Serves: 5
Preparation time: 10 minutes, plus chiling

½ cup very light cream cheese
heaping ⅓ cup fat-free Greek yogurt
4½oz smoked salmon, chopped
juice of ½ lemon
1 large dill sprig, chopped
freshly ground black pepper

1 Put all the ingredients in a blender or food processor and blend until smooth. Chill before serving.

Nutritional information per serving
Kcals 75 Protein **9g** Carbohydrate **2g** Fat **3g**

 Best for Cravings Hunger. Salmon is a great source of healthy omega-3 fats. These are known to improve attention span in children and can also reduce Cravings Hunger in adults by boosting focus and concentration to stick to a diet. Also good for 🥣 🥣 🥣 🥣 🥣 🥣

Red Pepper Dip

Sweet-tasting red bell peppers give this a lovely flavor as well as a great color.

Serves: 5
Preparation time: 5 minutes
Cooking time: 10 minutes, plus cooling and chiling

4 red bell peppers, cut in half and seeded
2 garlic cloves, crushed
1 teaspoon ground cumin
1 teaspoon Worcestershire sauce
juice of 1 lime
1 cup low-fat Greek yogurt
1 cup very light cream cheese

1 Preheat the broiler. Put the peppers on the broiler pan, skin-side up, and broil for 5–10 minutes until slightly blackened and starting to collapse. Remove from the broiler and put in a plastic bag to cool.
2 Remove from the bag and peel off the skin. Put the peppers and the other ingredients into a blender or food processor and blend until smooth. Chill before serving.

Nutritional information per serving
Kcals **63** Protein **17g** Carbohydrate **10g** Fat **4g**

Best for Anxious Hunger. Bell peppers are high in vitamin C, which is a co-factor for the production of the natural appetite-suppressant serotonin. They also contain natural sugars, which can help to potentiate serotonin's action. Also good for 🥣 🥣 🥣 🥣 🥣

Higher-Protein Hummus

This has the flavor of classic hummus, but is lower in fat and carbs.

Serves: 5
Preparation time: 10 minutes

scant 1 cup canned chickpeas, drained and rinsed
1 garlic clove, crushed
a squeeze of lime juice
1 teaspoon olive oil
4 tablespoons fat-free Greek yogurt
1 teaspoon ground cumin
a pinch of ground coriander
1 teaspoon chopped cilantro leaves
sea salt and freshly ground black pepper

1 Put all the ingredients into a blender or food processor and blend until smooth. Chill before serving.

Nutritional information per serving
Kcals **72** Protein **5g** Carbohydrate **21g** Fat **6g**

Best for Never-full Hunger. Estrogen is a fat-storage hormone. Chickpeas contain a weak form called phytoestrogens, which can block our cells' receptors for the stronger human form, reducing the overall estrogen load and so reducing fat storage. Also good for

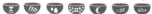

Mustardy Butter Bean Dip

If you like hummus, this is a creamy alternative. Butter beans are quite bland, so the mustard really gives this dip lots of flavor.

Serves: 5
Preparation time: 5 minutes, plus chilling

1 x 14oz can butter beans, drained and rinsed
2 tablespoons wholegrain mustard
juice of 2 lemons
sea salt and freshly ground black pepper

1 Put all the ingredients into a blender or food processor, and gradually add about ⅔ cup water while blending until you have a smooth, but not watery, dip. Chill before serving.

Nutritional information per serving
Kcals **65** Protein **5g** Carbohydrate **10g** Fat **2g**

Best for PMS Hunger. Butter beans are high in fiber, which is needed by the body to excrete toxins, including old hormones, and restore hormone balance. Unbalanced sex hormones can cause PMS-related overeating or exacerbate PCOS weight. Also good for

Warm Mexican Bean Dip

Chunky salsas are difficult to eat with vegetable sticks because the salsa falls off, but this one is blended to get round this problem.

Serves: 5
Preparation time: 10 minutes
Cooking time: 20 minutes, plus cooling

olive oil spray
1 onion, chopped
1 teaspoon white wine vinegar
1 garlic clove, crushed
1 dried chili, chopped
1 x 14oz can mixed beans, drained and rinsed
1 x 14oz can chopped tomatoes
1 teaspoon stevia-based granulated sweetener

1 Put a nonstick saucepan over medium heat and spray with oil, then fry the onion for 3–4 minutes until soft.
2 Add the vinegar, garlic and chili, and fry for 1 minute. Add the remaining ingredients and simmer for 10–15 minutes to reduce. Leave to cool slightly, then use a blender or food processor to blend until smooth. Serve the dip warm. (It is also excellent chilled.)

Nutritional information per serving
Kcals **76** Protein **9g** Carbohydrate **13g** Fat **2g**

 Best for Stress Hunger. Chili contains the compound capsaicin, which has been shown to improve blood sugar regulation. Stress can disrupt blood sugar, and unbalanced blood sugar causes cravings, mood swings and weight gain. Also good for

Spinach and Parmesan Dip

Here is an unusual veggie dip that also makes a great sauce for chicken or fish when served hot.

Serves: 5
Preparation time: 5 minutes
Cooking time: 5 minutes, plus cooling and chiling

olive oil spray
1lb spinach
1 cup fat-free Greek yogurt
½ cup freshly grated Parmesan cheese
4 scallions, chopped
1 garlic clove
juice of 1 lemon

1 Put a nonstick saucepan over medium heat and spray with oil, then gradually add the spinach, pressing it down and turning it over using tongs as it begins to wilt. Drain in a colander, then transfer to paper towels to absorb the remaining moisture, and leave to cool.
2 Put into a blender or food processor with all the other ingredients and blend until smooth. Chill before serving.

Nutritional information per serving
Kcals 86 Protein 9g Carbohydrate 15g Fat 3g

 Best for Tired Hunger. Spinach is high in energy-boosting iron and also contains magnesium, which the body needs to make the sleep hormone melatonin. Being tired or lacking in sleep both increase appetite. Also good for

All-Day Breakfast Eggs

Breakfast as a snack—sort of!

Serves: 2
Preparation time: 15 minutes
Cooking time: 10 minutes, plus cooling

2 eggs
1 slice Canadian bacon
½ teaspoon wholegrain mustard
2 teaspoons very light cream cheese

1 Put the eggs in a pan of boiling water and cook for 10 minutes. Drain the eggs and put them in a bowl of cold water to cool. Peel off the shells.
2 Meanwhile, preheat the broiler. Put the bacon on a broiler pan and broil until golden on both sides, turning over once. Cut into small pieces.
3 Cut the eggs in half and remove the yolks. Chop the yolks finely and put them in a small bowl. Add the mustard, cream cheese and half the bacon. Fill the centers of the egg whites with this mixture, and sprinkle the remaining bacon over the top. Serve.

Nutritional information per serving
Kcals **110** Protein **10g** Carbohydrate **trace** Fat **8g**

Best for Winter-Blues Hunger. Meat contains vitamin D, which we can make endogenously (that is, in our skin) when the sun shines. In winter, many of us are low in vitamin D and that can lead to depression and overeating. Also good for

Eggs Nicosia

Canned tuna basically tastes of cardboard, but if you add olives and anchovies, you suddenly have something very tasty indeed.

Serves: 2
Preparation time: 10 minutes
Cooking time: 10 minutes, plus cooling

2 eggs
⅓ cup canned tuna in spring water, drained
1 tablespoon fat-free Greek yogurt

¼ red onion, finely chopped
¼ celery stalk, finely chopped
1 canned anchovy, drained on paper towels, finely chopped (save the rest of the can for a meal)
1 tomato, chopped
2 pitted back olives, sliced into rings, to serve

1 Put the eggs in a pan of boiling water and cook for 10 minutes. Drain the eggs and put them in a bowl of cold water to cool. Peel off the shells.
2 Cut the eggs in half and remove the yolks. Chop the yolks finely and put them in a small bowl. Add the remaining ingredients. Mix well and use to fill the centers of the egg whites. Serve with the black olive slices on top.

Nutritional information per serving
Kcals **116** Protein **13g** Carbohydrate **6g** Fat **6g**

 Best for Cravings Hunger. Greek yogurt is a good source of calcium. This mineral has been shown to inhibit the hormone ghrelin, which switches on appetite. Also good for 🥣 🌙 💤 40+

Guacamole Eggs

This really does raise the humble boiled egg to new heights.

Serves: 2
Preparation time: 10 minutes
Cooking time: 10 minutes, plus
  cooling

2 eggs
¼ avocado, peeled, pitted and
  chopped

1 tomato, chopped
¼ fresh chili, seeded and chopped
a squeeze of lime juice
2 teaspoons chopped cilantro leaves
sea salt and freshly ground black
  pepper

1 Put the eggs in a pan of boiling water and cook for 10 minutes. Drain the eggs and put them in a bowl of cold water to cool. Peel off the shells.
2 Cut the eggs in half and remove the yolks. Chop the yolks finely and put them in a small bowl. Add the remaining ingredients and season with salt and pepper to taste. Mix well and use to fill the centers of the egg whites, then serve.

Nutritional information per serving
Kcals **111** Protein **7g** Carbohydrate **2g** Fat **9g**

Best for Emotional Hunger. Avocados contain tryptophan, which the body converts into the appetite-suppressing hormone serotonin. Also good for

FRUIT, NUTS AND SEEDS

Fruit

You will probably notice that there isn't much fruit in this book. Research on fructose is beginning to suggest that it might actually be more fattening than other sugars. Plus, dieters tend to see fruit as a "free" food, so they often overeat it. And, yes, fruit does contain valuable stuff like disease-fighting antioxidants, but sweet fruits such as banana, pineapple and mango can also maintain a sugar addiction, unbalancing blood sugar and causing weight gain.

All this means that I am not a big fan of fruit as a weight-loss snack; however, I have included a few suggestions that combine protein and/or healthy fats with the fruit to offset the sugar hit.

Nuts and seeds

With their combination of healthy fats and protein, nuts and seeds are a great snack *if* you can control your portion sizes. Before making any of these snacks, ask yourself the question: "Is an open bag of cashews an empty bag of cashews?" Seeds tend to be a bit less addictive than nuts and can be an easier choice. If you think you can control yourself, then make these snacks and put them into little bags. They are super-portable and super-healthy.

Melon and Ham Roll-Ups

This is a bit of a retro recipe, but no worse for that. It's sweet and salty.

Serves: 2
Preparation time: 5 minutes

3½oz melon
4 slices of dry-cured unsmoked ham, about 2½oz, fat removed

1 Cut the melon flesh from the skin, then cut the flesh into matchsticks.
Divide the melon between the four slices of ham, roll up and serve.

Nutritional information per serving
Kcals **90** Protein **11g** Carbohydrate **2g** Fat **1g**

Best for Tired Hunger. Melon is a medium-GI fruit, so it doesn't upset blood sugar. Plus, it contains vitamin C, which is needed to make the sleep hormone melatonin. A good night's sleep reduces appetite the following day. Also good for 🥣 🥣

Broiled Pear with Ricotta and Cinnamon

Here's a rather elegant snack with a lovely warm hint of cinnamon.

Serves: 2
Preparation time: 5 minutes
Cooking time: 10 minutes

2 pears, cut in half
4 tablespoons low-fat ricotta cheese
a pinch of ground cinnamon

1 Preheat the broiler to medium. Cut out the cores of the pear halves to make a slight cavity. Put the pear halves, skin-side down, on the broiler pan. Cook for 5–10 minutes until tender. Remove from the broiler.
2 Fill the cavities of the pears with the ricotta and sprinkle over the cinnamon, then serve.

Nutritional information per serving
Kcals **81** Protein **4g** Carbohydrate **11g** Fat **2g**

 Best for Cravings Hunger. Ricotta cheese is special in that of all cheeses it is the highest in the amino acid tyrosine. This is converted in the body to the cravings-fighting neurotransmitter dopamine. Also good for

Apple and Blue Cheese Melt

Sweet apple and salty blue cheese work really well, but you can choose goat's cheese or Cheddar, if you prefer.

Serves: 2
Preparation time: 10 minutes
Cooking time: 5 minutes

olive oil spray
2 apples, cored and thinly sliced
¼ cup crumbled blue cheese such as Stilton or Dolcelatte

1 Preheat the broiler to medium. Line the broiler pan with aluminum foil and spray with oil. Arrange the apple slices in two circles with the edges of the slices overlapping to form a base.
2 Sprinkle over the cheese and broil for 2–3 minutes to melt the cheese. Remove from the broiler and use a fish spatula to slide the melts out onto two plates. Serve.

Nutritional information per serving
Kcals **97** Protein **3g** Carbohydrate **11g** Fat **4g**

 Best for 40+ Hunger. Dairy foods such as cheese contain natural progesterone, which declines in women over 40 and can contribute to symptoms of mid-life depression and apple-shaped weight gain. Also good for

Tangy Sunflower Seeds

Love salted peanuts? This is a much healthier crunchy snack.

Serves: 5
Preparation time: 5 minutes
Cooking time: 10 minutes, plus cooling

1 tablespoon canola oil
2 tablespoons Worcestershire sauce
¾ cup sunflower seeds

1 Preheat the oven to 300ºF. Put the oil and Worcestershire sauce in a bowl
and mix together. Add the seeds and stir to combine.
2 Spread the seeds out on a baking sheet and roast for 10 minutes until
lightly toasted, being careful not to burn them. Leave the seeds to cool before
serving. Store in an airtight container for up to 1 month.

Nutritional information per serving
Kcals **103** Protein **15g** Carbohydrate **3g** Fat **9g**

Best for Tired Hunger, because sunflower seeds contain
B vitamins and iron, both of which help to boost
energy and so reduce tired overeating. Also good for

Spiced Almonds

My top three nutritious nuts are Brazils, walnuts and, as here, almonds. Smoked almonds (which I love) are usually too high in salt. These spiced almonds have a great flavor, but contain less salt. My recipe for the spice blend will give you extra to store and use for several batches of almonds.

Serves: 5
Preparation time: 10 minutes
Cooking time: 20 minutes, plus cooling

2 teaspoons canola oil
2 teaspoons spice blend (see right)
½ cup whole blanched almonds

For the spice blend
1 tablespoon sea salt
1 tablespoon garlic powder
1 tablespoon celery salt
1 tablespoon onion powder
1 tablespoon chili powder
2 tablespoons paprika
1 tablespoon stevia-based granulated sweetener
1 teaspoon dried sage
a pinch each of dried thyme, cayenne pepper, mustard powder and black pepper

1 Preheat the oven to 300°F. To make the spice blend, put all the ingredients in a bowl and mix well. Transfer to an airtight container and store for up to 1 month.
2 Put the oil and spice blend in a small bowl and mix well. Add the almonds and stir to coat completely in the spicy mix. Spread the almonds out on a baking sheet and roast for 15–20 minutes until lightly toasted, being careful not to burn them. Leave the nuts to cool before serving. Store in an airtight container for up to 1 month.

Nutritional information per serving
Kcals **198** Protein **3g** Carbohydrate **1g** Fat **10g**

Best for Anxious Hunger. All tree nuts (peanuts are a ground nut) are an excellent source of healthy fats, which make all our hunger hormones work efficiently. Almonds have the added bonus of containing glutamic acid, which our bodies need to make the anxiety-fighting brain hormone GABA. Also good for 🥣 🥣 🥣 🥣 🥣

Pepitas Calientes

Pumpkin seeds are used for this traditional Mexican snack. They have a fantastic mix of sweet, sour and hot flavors.

Serves: 5
Preparation time: 5 minutes
Cooking time: 5 minutes, plus cooling

½ cup pumpkin seeds
1 teaspoon garlic powder
1 teaspoon cayenne pepper
a pinch of sea salt
1 teaspoon stevia-based granulated sweetener
a squeeze of lime juice

1 Put the pumpkin seeds in a nonstick skillet and dry-fry for 2–3 minutes until they swell slightly but do not burn.
2 Add the other ingredients and stir to coat, then cook for 1 minute or until the liquid has evaporated. Leave the seeds to cool before serving. Store in an airtight container for up to 1 month.

Nutritional information per serving
Kcals **89** Protein **4g** Carbohydrate **11g** Fat **4g**

Best for 40+ Hunger. Pumpkin seeds are high in zinc, and this supports thyroid function, which can become less efficient as we get older. A sluggish thyroid means a slow metabolic rate, and this means you put on weight more easily. Also good for 🥣 🥣 🥣 🥣 🥣 🥣 🥣

SWEET THINGS

Frozen yogurt

I used to love ice cream—and I would eat it by the tub. These days I eat frozen yogurt, although not often the stuff you buy in supermarkets. The reason? It's full of sugar, and it is not as slimming as you might think. You're far better off making your own sugar-free versions at home to eat as a delicious snack.

Sweet bites

I am not a big fan of fruit as a weight-loss snack, but I have come up with a few suggestions in the book. In this section the fruit is combined with a healthy fat (lemon with coconut) to offset the fructose hit, slow down the blood sugar spike and keep you stable.

One last little chocolate treat! I like to put at least one chocolate recipe in every diet book (this one has several!). This isn't to trip you up but to show you that you can have chocolate and lose weight.

Vanilla Frozen Yogurt

This is simple – just three ingredients – but as with all simple recipes, technique is all. It is smoothest if made in an ice-cream maker.

Serves: 8
Preparation time: 5 minutes, plus 20 minutes in an ice-cream maker/ 3¾ hours in a freezer, plus 20 minutes defrosting

4½ cups fat-free Greek yogurt, chilled
⅔ cup agave syrup
1 teaspoon vanilla extract

1 Put all the ingredients in an ice-cream maker and churn until frozen. Alternatively, put the ingredients in a bowl and stir together to combine. Transfer to a freezerproof container and freeze for 45 minutes or until the mixture starts to freeze around the edges.
2 Beat the mixture with a fork or a hand-held electric mixer. Put the container back into the freezer for another 2–3 hours until solid. Transfer to the fridge 20 minutes before serving to soften slightly.

Nutritional information per serving
Kcals **124** Protein **10g** Carbohydrate **20g** Fat **trace**

Best for Cravings Hunger. The milk from which yogurt is made contains the amino acid tyrosine, and our bodies convert this into dopamine, which helps to fight food cravings. Also good for

Chocolate Frozen Yogurt

Yes, it had to be done!

Serves: 8
Preparation time: 5 minutes, plus
20 minutes in an ice-cream
maker/3¾ hours in a freezer, plus
20 minutes defrosting

3 cups fat-free Greek yogurt
scant 1½ cups skim milk
½ cup agave syrup
3 tablespoons cocoa powder

1 Put all the ingredients in a bowl and stir together to combine. Transfer to an ice-cream maker and churn until frozen. Alternatively, transfer the mixture to a freezerproof container and freeze for 45 minutes or until the mixture starts to freeze around the edges.
2 Beat the mixture with a fork or a hand-held electric mixer. Put the container back into the freezer for another 2–3 hours until solid. Transfer to the fridge 20 minutes before serving to soften slightly.

Nutritional information per serving
Kcals **130** Protein **10g** Carbohydrate **18g** Fat **1g**

Best for Never-Full Hunger. Cocoa in chocolate is a good source of the mineral zinc. This has been shown to be low in those who have leptin resistance, which can drive Cravings and Never-Full Hunger. Also good for

Fastest-Ever Berry Frozen Yogurt

This is my standby recipe for when I want something sweet, NOW! OK, this isn't quite frozen yogurt, as it hasn't been churned, but it's much, much quicker. This recipe is only for two servings, because if you're going to freeze it, you're better off making "proper" frozen yogurt using the recipe on page 290 and simply adding the berries to that.

Serves: 2
Preparation time: 5 minutes

generous ¾ cup fat-free Greek yogurt
¾ cup frozen mixed berries
2 tablespoon stevia-based granulated
   sweetener

1 Put all the ingredients into a blender or food processor. Process until smooth and serve.

Nutritional information per serving
Kcals **69** Protein **8g** Carbohydrate **8g** Fat **trace**

Best for Winter-Blues Hunger. Berries are not only high in disease-fighting antioxidants but also the little seeds in them make them high in fiber as well. This helps you feel full, which can reduce the desire for winter comfort eating. Also good for ⬜ ⬜ ⬜

Candied Lemons with Coconut

Dried fruit can set off sugar cravings in many, but choosing lemons, and the zest to boot, makes these candied lemons a lower GI, but still a lovely treat.

Serves: 8
Preparation time: 15 minutes
Baking time: 4¼ hours

4 tablespoon stevia-based granulated
  sweetener
juice of 2 limes
8 lemons, zest pared into strips
  (see Tip)
1¼ cups shredded coconut

1 Preheat the oven to 200°F. Put 1 generous cup water in a medium saucepan over medium heat and add the sweetener and lime juice. Heat through until the sweetener has dissolved. Add the zest, and bring to a boil, then reduce the heat and simmer, uncovered, for 15 minutes.
2 Line a baking sheet with parchment paper. Spread out the lemon zest. Pour over the remaining syrup and sprinkle with the coconut. Bake for 3–4 hours until the peel is sticky rather than downright crispy, and definitely not burned. If necessary, cover loosely with a piece of aluminum foil to avoid overbrowning. Remove from the oven and allow to cool before serving. Store in an airtight container for up to 2 weeks.

Tip: Use a vegetable peeler to take off just the zest in strips, leaving the bitter pith behind.

Nutritional information per serving
Kcals **54** Protein **0.5g** Carbohydrate **4g** Fat **4g**

Best for PMS Hunger. A compound in lemon zest has been shown to support liver function. This may improve detoxification, rebalance hormones and reduce hormonally driven weight gain. Also good for 🥣 🥣 🥣 🥣

Chocolate and Hazelnut Thins
with Sea Salt

OK, this is a last little treat. It isn't on any of the Food Plans, because it's not strictly a diet recipe. It's a lovely indulgence instead. The important thing is you can eat (a little) chocolate and lose weight as long as you avoid the sweet, milky kind (sorry!) and opt instead for high cocoa-content dark chocolate (look for at least 70 percent cocoa solids on the pack). It's richer, so it's less easy to binge on, but it will still give you that cocoa hit. If you think it will set you off on a chocolate roller coaster, however, choose another snack.

Serves: 8
Preparation time: 15 minutes
Cooking time: 15 minutes, plus cooling and chiling

heaping ⅓ cup chopped hazelnuts
1 teaspoon stevia-based granulated sweetener
4½ oz dark chocolate (70% cocoa solids), roughly chopped
coarse sea salt, to sprinkle

1 Preheat the oven to 350°F. Spread the nuts on a baking sheet and bake for 5 minutes or until golden, but not burned. Sprinkle with the sweetener and bake for another 1 minute. Leave the nuts to cool.
2 Put the chocolate in a heatproof bowl over a saucepan of gently simmering water, making sure the base of the bowl doesn't touch the water. Leave the chocolate to melt very gently, stirring it as little as possible.
3 Line a baking sheet with parchment paper. When the chocolate has melted, drop 16 spoonfuls onto the paper, allowing them to spread into little discs. Sprinkle with the nuts and sea salt, then transfer to the fridge to chill until firm. Carefully remove the chocolates from the parchment paper and store in an airtight container in the fridge before serving. They will store for up to 1 month.

Chocolate and Lemon Thins *Follow the recipe above, but omit the hazelnuts and sea salt and replace with ⅓ cup very finely chopped Candied Lemons with Coconut (see page 293).*

Chocolate and Ginger Thins *Follow the recipe above, but omit the hazelnuts and sea salt. Drain 3 balls stem ginger from a jar and pat off as much sugar syrup as you can using paper towels. Chop the ginger very finely. This isn't quite as low in sugar as the lemon recipe above, but it is a lovely treat.*

A word about chocolate

I have tried making the above with sugar-free chocolate and it works, but it just doesn't taste as good. Sugar-free dark chocolate has a greasy taste, to me, and doesn't deliver the same hit of cocoa solids. I think you're better off eating a smaller amount of really great dark chocolate. My preference is Lindt, although Green & Black's and Divine are good too. Another excellent chocolate is Ghirardelli intense dark gourmet bar.

Nutritional information per serving
Kcals **120** Protein **2g** Carbohydrate **9g** Fat **10g**

Best for Cravings Hunger. Chocolate has enough feel-good compounds in it to fill a chemistry lab—sugar, caffeine and l-phenylalanine to name but three. But certain Hunger Typers really should avoid it. For anxious or stress eaters, it can trigger both migraines and hyperactivity. It can also set Hedonistic eaters off on a binge. Also good for

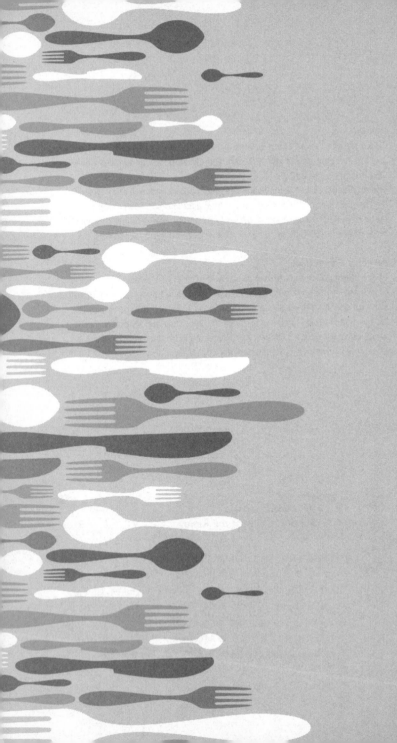

Main Meals

It's a scenario familiar to many of us. You've been "good" all day and then as soon as evening comes it all falls apart. You graze your way through the fridge while you're cooking dinner, you eat your dinner (although you're not really that hungry any more) and then you spend the rest of the evening searching for little snacks like a snuffly, chocolate-truffle pig.

So, how to avoid that? First, of course, is to identify the kind of hunger that is driving this behavior. Hopefully, you've already done that by completing the Quiz on pages 94–7. Next, choose food that addresses your hunger type *and* is quick and easy. The last bit is really important, because there's no point in deciding on a great supper if you have to be Gordon Ramsay to cook it.

The Hunger Type dinner recipes are designed to be easy. They run from quick salads, stir-fries and even burgers, to curries and slow-cook casseroles. One of the main differences between my recipes and what you may have been eating is that starchy foods—rice, potatoes, pasta—are portion controlled or swapped for alternative, but more healthy, grains such as quinoa and barley.

In my experience, a bit of forward planning goes a long way when you're trying to lose weight. Finding you have no food in the house and that the only shop nearby is the gas station convenience store is not a good recipe for weight loss, in my opinion. Many of these Hunger Type Diet dinner recipes can be batch cooked (a real Sunday night job, this), then portioned up and either put in the fridge or the freezer. Then, you just reheat one when you need it. How simple is that?

I've included some recipes for entertaining too. When you're on a diet, you can feel like Billy No Mates. You turn down invitations to go out to dinner for fear of being tempted by the tiramisu, or you go and sit glumly with a glass of water and a green salad (no dressing). Even dinner at a friend's can be a trial, as either you have to make a show of yourself turning down food or you eat the lasagne and the cream puffs and then the scales tell the story afterwards.

The entertaining section features slightly more complicated recipes that still fit the Hunger Type Food Plan, so you can cook for others while remaining on track. Yes, you can lose weight and have friends too!

LIGHT MEALS

Salad mains

Some may see salad as a lunch dish, but these salads are substantial, featuring a hot main event on a bed of leaves. The benefit of making a salad, rather than cooking vegetables, is that all you have to do is arrange it, so it speeds things up.

Supper on a tray

When I was a child, I loved spaghetti hoops on toast on a tray in front of the TV. It was so fantastically comforting. I'm not going to suggest that as a nutritionally balanced meal (hey, I was brought up in the era of crinkle-cut chips and Vienetta), but the combination of toast and tray has an emotional connection with homeyness and comfort for many of us. Here are some ideas for when you just want some supper to curl up with.

Burgers

For a really speedy supper, burgers are good because you can make them in advance and they cook quickly; however, the traditional burger staple—ground beef—is high in fat and calories. Here are some ideas using turkey, tuna, tofu and beans. None of these burgers is designed to go in a bun. Add steamed veggies or a simple leaf salad.

Dinnertime eggs

Nutritious eggs cook in a flash and are high in protein, so they help you feel full. As for worries about cholesterol, the best medical advice now is that it's not how much cholesterol you eat but how you process it that matters. Although eggs may contain cholesterol, unless your doctor has specifically told you to avoid cholesterol-containing foods, there is no need to worry.

Some people can be allergic to eggs, particularly if they suddenly start eating a lot of them. If you feel constipated or have other digestive symptoms, swap to something else for a while.

Tamarind-Glazed Chicken Salad

The slightly sour tang of tamarind complements the chicken beautifully.

Serves: 2
Preparation time: 15 minutes, plus
2 hours marinating
Cooking time: 10 minutes

2 skinless chicken breasts, 4¼oz each
olive oil spray

For the ginger-tamarind marinade
1 tablespoon tamarind paste
¾-inch piece of ginger root, peeled
and grated
1 garlic clove, crushed
a pinch of sea salt
a pinch of ground cumin
2 teaspoons agave syrup

For the tamarind dressing
2 teaspoons tamarind paste
2 teaspoons Thai fish sauce
2 teaspoons soy sauce
juice of ½ lime
2 teaspoons stevia-based granulated
sweetener
½ red chili, seeded and finely sliced

For the salad
1 romaine lettuce, separated into
leaves
1 cucumber, sliced
8 radishes, finely sliced
1 red onion, finely sliced

1 Start preparations in the morning. Put the chicken between two pieces of plastic wrap and use a rolling pin or the base of a skillet to bash it to about ½-inch thick. Put the marinade ingredients in a small bowl and mix well.
2 Put the chicken in a shallow dish, then pour over the marinade and mix to coat the chicken completely. Cover the dish and chill for at least 2 hours.
3 Put the dressing ingredients in a screw-topped jar and shake. Put a griddle pan over medium-high heat and spray with oil. Cook the chicken for 3 minutes on each side until cooked. Serve with the salad and dressing.

Nutritional information per serving
Kcals **257** Protein **33g** Carbohydrate **29g** Fat **2g**

Best for Tired Hunger. A high-sugar meal can make you feel tired. Here, sugar is replaced with agave syrup, which has a lower GI, thus preventing the post-meal slump that can fuel tired overeating. Also good for

Vietnamese Shaking-Beef Salad

This is a light version of the Vietnamese classic.

Serves: 2
Preparation time: 10 minutes, plus 4 hours marinating
Cooking time: 5 minutes

1 tablespoon soy sauce
1 tablespoon Thai fish sauce
2 garlic cloves, crushed
2 teaspoons stevia-based granulated sweetener

1 teaspoon sesame oil
7oz filet mignon, cut into small chunks
olive oil spray

For the salad
7oz watercress
1 romaine lettuce, separated into leaves
1 red onion, thinly sliced

1 Start preparations in the morning. Put the soy sauce in a small bowl and add the fish sauce, garlic, sweetener and sesame oil. Mix together well. Put the beef in a shallow dish and pour over the mixture, then mix to coat the beef completely. Cover the dish and chill for at least 4 hours.

2 Put a nonstick skillet over medium heat and spray with oil. Drain the beef, reserving the marinade, and add the beef to the pan. Cook over medium-high heat for 2–3 minutes, then add the marinade and heat through. Put the salad on serving plates and serve with the beef.

Nutritional information per serving
Kcals **341** Protein **39g** Carbohydrate **13g** Fat **12g**

Best for Hedonistic Hunger. The protein and fat in red meat slows down stomach emptying, helping you feel full and preventing overeating. Also good for

Cod and Lychee Salad with Miso Dressing

The classic miso fish is cod, as suggested here, but you can substitute any firm white fish such as pollock or tilapia.

Serves: 2

Preparation time: 15 minutes, plus 24 hours marinating

Cooking time: 11 minutes, plus cooling

4 cod fillets, or other white fish fillets, 4¼oz each

olive oil spray

scant ½ cup shredded fresh coconut (optional)

For the miso dressing

2 tablespoons sake

2 tablespoons mirin

½ cup white miso paste

2 tablespoons stevia-based granulated sweetener

For the salad

3½ oz arugula (about 3–4 cups)

1 oak leaf lettuce, separated into leaves

4 fresh lychees, peeled, pitted and thinly sliced

1 small bunch of cilantro leaves, chopped

1 Start preparations the day before. To make the dressing, put the sake and mirin in a small saucepan over medium heat. Boil for 30 seconds to burn off the alcohol. Reduce the heat and add the miso paste and sweetener. Stir to dissolve. Remove from the heat and leave to cool.

2 Put the fish in a shallow dish. Pour half the dressing over and mix to coat completely. Cover and chill for 24 hours. Reserve the remaining dressing.

3 Preheat the broiler and the oven to 400°F. Remove the cod from the dressing and wipe off the dressing. Spray a broiler pan with oil and lay the fish in the pan. Broil for 2–3 minutes, then transfer the broiler pan to the oven for 5–8 minutes until the fish is cooked through.

4 Put the salad ingredients on serving plates, top with the fish, then drizzle with the reserved miso dressing. Sprinkle with coconut, if using. Serve.

Nutritional information per serving
Kcals **303** Protein **31g** Carbohydrate **25g** Fat **10g**

Best for Never-Full Hunger. Fish and seafood are a source of zinc, which may improve leptin resistance, switching off hunger. Also good for

Red Mullet, Almond and Fennel Salad with a Blood Orange Dressing

This is a very elegant salad with a slightly sweet dressing.

Serves: 2
Preparation time: 15 minutes
Cooking time: 20 minutes, plus cooling

olive oil spray
2 red mullet or snapper fillets, 4¼oz each
1 egg white, lightly beaten
scant ⅔ cups slivered almonds

For the blood orange dressing
juice of 4 blood oranges
1 star anise
2 green cardamom pods
½ teaspoon fennel seeds
1 tablespoon olive oil
juice of 1 lemon

For the salad
½ head of radicchio, separated into leaves
1 packed cup watercress
½ fennel bulb, thinly sliced

1 To make the dressing, pour the orange juice into a small saucepan over medium heat and bring to a boil, then reduce the heat and simmer for 5 minutes until reduced by two-thirds. Add the star anise, cardamom and fennel seeds, and cook for 2 minutes. Remove from the heat and leave to cool. Pour through a sieve into a bowl, then beat in the oil and lemon juice.
2 Preheat the broiler and spray the broiler pan with oil. Dip the skin side of the fish in the egg white and coat it in the almonds. Put it in the broiler pan, skin-side up, and broil for 8–10 minutes until cooked through. Put the salad on plates and serve with the fish and a drizzle of the dressing.

Nutritional information per serving
Kcals **480** Protein **33g** Carbohydrate **24g** Fat **30g**

Best for Anxious Hunger. Fennel is a prebiotic food (it feeds probiotic bacteria in your gut), which is needed to make the anti-anxiety hormone GABA. Also good for

Scallop and Green Papaya Salad

In Asian cooking, green papaya is cooked as a vegetable. You can buy it in Asian supermarkets, and they also sell special peelers to make the super-fine matchsticks. Otherwise, just use a sharp knife and cut the matchsticks as thinly as possible.

Serves: 2
Preparation time: 15 minutes
Cooking time: 1 minute

¼ fresh green papaya, peeled, seeded and cut into matchsticks
4 scallions, sliced
2 carrots, peeled and grated
½ green cabbage, shredded
2 tablespoons chopped mint leaves
2 tablespoons chopped cilantro leaves
2 tablespoons chopped Thai basil leaves
8 shelled sea scallops, 5¾oz total weight
olive oil spray

For the ginger and chili dressing
1 tablespoon stevia-based granulated sweetener
juice of ½ lime
½ garlic clove, crushed
½-inch piece of ginger root, peeled and grated
1 teaspoon Thai fish sauce
1 red chili, seeded and finely chopped
1 teaspoon sesame oil

1 Put a griddle pan over medium-high heat. Meanwhile, put the dressing ingredients in a screw-topped jar and shake well.
2 Put the papaya in a bowl and add the scallions, carrots, cabbage and herbs, then pour in the dressing. Toss together to coat well.
3 Spray both sides of the scallops with oil and put in the griddle pan for 20–30 seconds each side. Serve the scallops with the salad.

Nutritional information per serving
Kcals **258** Protein **22g** Carbohydrate **20g** Fat **8g**

Best for Emotional Hunger, because papaya contains the antidepressant ingredient tryptophan. Also good for

Puy Lentil Salad with Goat Cheese and Rosewater Dressing

This is a filling salad with an interestingly spicy, but scented, dressing.

Serves: 2
Preparation time: 20 minutes
Cooking time: 20 minutes

⅓ cup dried Puy lentils
1 small bunch broccoli, cut into flore
¼ cup pine nuts
2 packed cups watercress
¼ cup crumbled goat's cheee

For the rosewater dressing
2 teaspoons wholegrain mustard
2 teaspoons ground coriander
2 teaspoons ground cumin
2 teaspoons ground cinnamon
1 teaspoon agave syrup
2 teaspoons white wine vinegar
1 tablespoon olive oil
2 teaspoons rosewater
1 handful of mint leaves, chopped
1 handful of parsley leaves, chopped
sea salt and freshly ground black
    pepper

1 To make the dressing, put the mustard, spices and agave syrup into a mini food processor and blend until smooth. While still blending, gradually add the vinegar, oil and rosewater until emulsified. Add the mint and parsley, and season to taste with salt and pepper, then set aside.

2 Put the lentils in a large saucepan over high heat and add twice the volume of boiling water. Bring to a boil and cook for 15–20 minutes until soft, adding the broccoli florets for the last 5 minutes. Drain in a colander, then return the mixture to the pan.

3 Meanwhile, put the pine nuts in a small saucepan and toast over medium heat until golden, tossing the pan frequently and being careful not to burn them. Set aside. Stir the dressing into the lentils. Serve the dressed lentils on the watercress with the pine nuts and goat's cheese on top.

> **Nutritional information per serving**
> Kcals **398** Protein **41g** Carbohydrate **43g** Fat **33g**

 Best for Stress Hunger. Many people overeat at night to try to de-stress themselves. Lentils can help, because they contain glutamic acid, which converts into GABA, the anti-anxiety hormone. Also good for 🥣 🥣 🥣 🌙 40+

Better BLT

Why's it better? Because I've dumped most of the fat from the bacon and the greasy mayo. Once you've done that, and added some really good bread, the humble BLT becomes actually rather good for you.

Serves: 2
Preparation time: 5 minutes
Cooking time: 5 minutes

6 slices unsmoked Canadian bacon

4 slices Chickpea and Rosemary Bread (see page 254)
2 teaspoons very light cream cheese
4 lettuce leaves
1 tomato, thinly sliced

1 Preheat the broiler. Put the bacon on a broiler pan and broil until golden on both sides, turning over once.
2 Spread the bread with the cream cheese, then top two slices with a lettuce leaf. Divide the bacon between the two lettuce leaves and put the sliced tomato on top. Finish with the remaining lettuce and another slice of bread, then serve.

Nutritional information per serving
Kcals 375 Protein 21g Carbohydrate 7g Fat 16g

 Best for PMS Hunger, because red meat is a source of iron. This can lift energy, offsetting the tiredness that can be a factor in PMS. Also good for

Posh Sardines on Toast

This is a Spanish take on classic beans on toast with tomatoes, spices and chickpeas. It's so much nicer than just opening a can.

Serves: 2
Preparation time: 10 minutes
Cooking time: 12 minutes

olive oil spray
½ onion, finely chopped
1 red bell pepper, seeded and thinly sliced
a pinch of paprika
a pinch of ground cinnamon

½ cup canned chickpeas, drained and rinsed
juice of 1 lemon
1 handful of parsley leaves, chopped
1 lemon, sliced
2 fresh sardines, cleaned
2 thin slices of Rye and Fennel Seed Bread (see page 211) or 4 slices of whole-wheat bread

1 Preheat the broiler to medium-high and spray the broiler pan with oil. Put a nonstick saucepan over medium heat and spray with oil, then fry the onion for 5 minutes or until soft. Add the red bell pepper and cook for another 1 minute, then stir in the paprika and cinnamon (add a splash of water if the mixture sticks to the pan).

2 Add the chickpeas and lemon juice, and cook for 1–2 minutes to warm through. Take off the heat and stir in the parsley.

3 Put the lemon slices inside the sardines and put them on the broiler for 4–5 minutes, turning once, until cooked through. Meanwhile, toast the bread. Put the toast on two plates and top with the chickpea mixture, then the sardines. Serve.

Nutritional information per serving
Kcals **424** Protein **34g** Carbohydrate **57g** Fat **9g**

 Best for Anxious Hunger. The oils in sardines may reduce histamine levels, thereby helping Anxious Hunger. Although there has been concern about mercury pollution in oily fish, this isn't a reason to avoid it. Remember that the bigger the fish, the more mercury, so small fish like sardines are a safer bet. Also good for 🥣 🥣 🥣 🥣 🥣

Poached Eggs and Asparagus on Toast

Egg on toast is a classic combination. Adding the asparagus just elevates it to something more sophisticated.

Serves: 2
Preparation time: 10 minutes
Cooking time: 5 minutes

8 asparagus spears
4 eggs
2 slices of Spelt and Seed Loaf (see page 252)
 or two thin slices of whole-wheat bread
sea salt and freshly ground black pepper

1 Snap off any woody ends from the asparagus stalks at the point where they break easily. Pour boiling water into a skillet to a depth of 1½ inches and return to a boil over medium-high heat. Put the asparagus spears in the pan and leave for 30 seconds then lift them out using tongs and transfer them to a colander. Refresh the asparagus under cold water and drain well.
2 Crack the eggs, one at a time, into the water, keeping them spaced apart if possible. Cook for 3–4 minutes each or until done to your liking. Meanwhile, toast the bread.
3 Separate the poached eggs using the edge of a slotted spoon and lift them out, then put them on paper towels to drain. Put the toast on two plates with the asparagus on top, then add the eggs, season and serve.

Nutritional information per serving
Kcals **325** Protein **21g** Carbohydrate **5g** Fat **14g**

Best for 40+ Hunger. Asparagus is high in the mineral potassium, which buffers too much sodium (salt) in the body. This helps with weight loss, because salt makes you retain water. Asparagus can therefore reduce bloating. Also good for 🥧 🥣 ❄️

Turkey and Feta Burgers

Adding feta cheese to these burgers keeps them moist and gives them a lovely hit of tanginess when you bite into them.

Serves: 2
Preparation time: 15 minutes, plus 30 minutes chiling
Cooking time: 10 minutes

1 cup chopped turkey breast
¾ cup crumbled feta cheese

1 bunch of parsley, leaves only
1 bunch of basil, leaves only
zest of 1 lemon
2 tablespoons whole-wheat flour
olive oil spray
freshly ground black pepper

1 Put all the ingredients, except the flour and oil spray, in a food processor. Season with pepper, and process to combine. Form into two balls, then put them on a plate and flatten them. Dust with the flour and chill them in the fridge for at least 30 minutes.
2 Put a nonstick skillet over medium-high heat and spray with oil. Fry the burgers for 4–5 minutes on each side to cook through thoroughly. Serve.

Nutritional information per serving
Kcals **271** Protein **27g** Carbohydrate **11g** Fat **11g**

 Best for PMS Hunger. Feta cheese is made from sheep's, not cow's, milk. Although cow's milk can be allergenic, causing bloating, swapping to sheep's milk products can reduce water retention and help you lose weight. Bloating is common premenstrually. Also good for

Spiced Tuna Burgers

Fresh tuna works just as well as meat to make a burger, although you do need breadcrumbs to lighten the mix.

Serves: 2
Preparation time: 15 minutes, plus 30 minutes chiling
Cooking time: 10 minutes

9oz fresh tuna, roughly chopped
2 shallots, finely chopped
1 egg white
1¾ cups fresh whole-wheat bread crumbs
1 tablespoon chopped mint leaves
1 teaspoon ground cumin
olive oil spray
sea salt and freshly ground black pepper

1 Put all the ingredients, except the oil spray, in a food processor. Season with salt and pepper, then process to combine. Form into two balls, then put them on a plate, flatten them and chill them in the fridge for at least 30 minutes.

2 Put a nonstick skillet over medium heat and spray with oil. Fry the burgers for 4–5 minutes on each side to cook through thoroughly. Serve.

Nutritional information per serving
Kcals **301** Protein **34g** Carbohydrate **28g** Fat **3g**

Best for Cravings Hunger. Mint is a good source of manganese, which is needed to make all the Hunger Type hormones, including the anti-cravings neurotransmitter dopamine. One of the lesser-known minerals, manganese can aid weight loss because it plays a vital role in fat and protein metabolism. Also good for

Butter Bean, Parmesan and Thyme Burgers

Creamy butter beans give a good texture to these burgers, but you do need to add plenty of flavor. Cheese and thyme are a really good combination.

Serves: 2
Preparation time: 15 minutes, plus 30 minutes chiling
Cooking time: 10 minutes

1 tablespoon olive oil
1¼ cups canned butter beans, drained and rinsed
½ onion, chopped
1 garlic clove, crushed
½ cup freshly grated Parmesan cheese
1 teaspoon thyme leaves
olive oil spray
sea salt and freshly ground black pepper

1 Put all the ingredients, except the oil spray, in a food processor. Season with salt and pepper, then process to combine. Form into two balls, then put them on a plate, flatten them and chill them in the fridge for at least 30 minutes.
2 Put a nonstick skillet over medium-high heat and spray with oil. Fry the burgers for 4–5 minutes on each side to cook through thoroughly. Serve.

Nutritional information per serving
Kcals **272** Protein **14g** Carbohydrate **26g** Fat **7g**

Best for Hedonistic Hunger. Butter beans are a source of zinc, which has been shown to be low in those with leptin resistence. Leptin should switch off appetite, but when you are resistant it doesn't. Increasing zinc might help. Also good for

Tofu and Beet Burgers

The beets give this burger a good color and keep it moist.

Serves: 2
Preparation time: 20 minutes, plus
  30 minutes chiling
Cooking time: 15 minutes

olive oil spray
1 onion, chopped
1 cup chopped button mushrooms
14oz firm tofu, drained and finely
  chopped

1 cup grated cooked beets (not in
  vinegar)
½ carrot, peeled and grated
⅔ cup canned kidney beans, drained,
  rinsed and chopped
1 teaspoon smoked paprika
1 garlic clove, crushed
sea salt and freshly ground black
  pepper

1 Put a nonstick saucepan over medium heat and spray with oil, then fry the onion for 2 minutes. Add the mushrooms and fry for 5 minutes. Transfer the mixture to a mixing bowl and leave to cool.
2 Drain off any liquid, then add the other ingredients, season with salt and pepper, and mix to combine. Form into two balls, then put them on a plate, flatten them and chill them in the fridge for at least 30 minutes.
3 Put a nonstick skillet over medium-high heat and spray with oil. Fry the burgers for 3–4 minutes on each side to cook through thoroughly. Serve.

Nutritional information per serving
Kcals **241** Protein **20g** Carbohydrate **22g** Fat **9g**

Best for Tired Hunger, because beets are a good source of energy-giving iron, which can help reduce tired eating. Also good for 🥣 🥣 🥣 🥣 🥣 🥣

Poached Eggs with Edamame and Kale

This recipe contains not one, not two, but three nutritional superstars: eggs, edamame (soybeans) and kale are all fantastic for you. Plus, it tastes great.

Serves: 2
Preparation time: 15 minutes
Cooking time: 6 minutes

½ medium head cauliflower, roughly chopped
olive oil spray

2 garlic cloves, sliced
a pinch of dried chili flakes
9oz kale, chopped
heaping ¾ cup fresh podded edamame beans
2 eggs
sea salt

1 Put the cauliflower into a food processor and process until the consistency of rice. Set aside. Put a large nonstick saucepan over medium heat and spray with oil, then cook the garlic and chili flakes for 1 minute, being careful not to burn them.

2 Add the cauliflower and kale, and cook for 2 minutes, stirring. Add the edamame and a splash of water, then cover and cook for 3 minutes to thoroughly heat the mixture through.

3 Meanwhile, pour boiling water into a skillet to a depth of 1½ inches and return to a boil over medium-high heat. Crack the eggs, one at a time, into the water, keeping them spaced apart if possible. Cook for 3–4 minutes each or until done to your liking. Lift out the eggs using a slotted spoon and put them on paper towels to drain. Serve the eggs on the kale mixture sprinkled with a little salt.

Nutritional information per serving
Kcals **300** Protein **15g** Carbohydrate **18g** Fat **11g**

Best for 40+ Hunger. The classic LA diet meal is the egg-white omelet, but it's the yolks that contain all the important fat-soluble vitamins. Egg yolks contain the antidepressant vitamin D and progesterone, which might help reduce the fat-storage effects of estrogen in the body. Also good for 🍸 🍳 🌙

Turkish Eggs with Tomato and Garlic Yogurt

My 11-year-old son recently announced that in my dream house I should have a room completely filled with yogurt, as I eat so much. So, I make no apology for including it A LOT in this book. As here, it's a fast way to add low-fat protein to a dish and it gives a fantastic, silky consistency too.

Serves: 2
Preparation time: 10 minutes
Cooking time: 20 minutes

olive oil spray
1 onion, sliced
1½ garlic cloves, crushed

1 red chili, seeded and chopped
1 x 14oz can chopped tomatoes
a pinch of stevia-based granulated sweetener
4 eggs
4 tablespoons fat-free Greek yogurt
2 tablespoons chopped parsley leaves

1 Put a nonstick skillet over medium heat and spray with oil, then fry the onion for 5 minutes or until soft. Add 1 garlic clove and the chili to the pan, and fry for 1 minute (add a splash of water if the mixture sticks to the pan). Add the tomatoes and sweetener, and simmer to reduce the mixture to a thick sauce.

2 Make 4 wells in the sauce and crack an egg into each. Cover with a lid or a layer of aluminum foil and cook for 3–4 minutes until the eggs are just set or done to your liking.

3 Meanwhile, put the yogurt in a bowl and beat in the parsley and remaining garlic. Serve the tomato and egg mixture with a dollop of the garlic yogurt on the top.

Nutritional information per serving
Kcals **254** Protein **18g** Carbohydrate **15g** Fat **10g**

 Best for Anxious Hunger. Garlic has a natural blood-thinning effect. This can lower blood pressure, which can help to offset anxious eating. Also good for

Mediterranean Eggs

Rather than frying eggs and then adding a side of vegetables, this recipe cooks the eggs in the veggies, so you get more flavor and less washing up!

Serves: 2
Preparation time: 10 minutes
Cooking time: 12 minutes

olive oil spray
2 large zucchinis, cut into
  ½-inch cubes

7oz cherry tomatoes,
  cut in half
1 garlic clove, crushed
4 eggs
1 handful of basil leaves
sea salt and freshly ground black
  pepper

1 Put a nonstick skillet over medium heat and spray with oil, then fry the zucchini for 5 minutes to soften them (add a splash of water if the mixture sticks to the pan). Add the tomatoes and garlic, and cook for 2 minutes.
2 Season with salt and pepper, then make 4 wells in the mixture and crack an egg into each. Cover with a lid or a layer of aluminum foil and cook for 3–4 minutes until the eggs are done to your liking. Serve scattered with basil leaves.

Nutritional information per serving
Kcals **218** Protein **17g** Carbohydrate **6g** Fat **20g**

Best for Stress Hunger. Basil is a traditional cure for stomach aches, migraines and anxiety. These same anti-spasmodic and muscle-relaxant properties make it helpful for reducing anxious and stress eating.
Also good for 🍴 🥣 🥣 ❄ 60+

DINNER AT THE TABLE

Proper dinners

For those who eat breakfast on the run and lunch at their desk, dinner is precious as the one meal that can be eaten properly—at a table. Here are a few recipes for what I call "proper dinners."

There are plenty of hearty casseroles and stews here. The great thing about these is that once you've got them going, you can just leave them to do their own thing. This is especially true if you have a slow cooker. All these stew recipes work in an oven or a slow cooker, but if you've never owned a slow cooker, you should seriously think about getting one, as it makes one-pot meals really easy. Cheaper cuts of meat are ideal, as slow cooking tenderizes them, and beans also taste great cooked this way. I've done all these recipes to serve four, so you can batch cook and have some ready-made suppers in the freezer.

As fish and seafood don't taste great cooked for hours in a crockpot—either going tough or disintegrating into a sticky puddle—I've included a few different recipes for fish, which are quick and simple to prepare after a long day at work.

Entertaining

There are times when you want to cook something a bit special. Here, you will find some showstopper dishes that are perfect for entertaining. I've created them to serve four, but you can reduce this if you're planning a more romantic dinner *à deux*.

Chicken Jalfrezi

Jalfrezis are hot, tomato-based curries, but if you prefer yours milder, just reduce the amount of chili.

Serves: 4
Preparation time: 10 minutes
Cooking time: 2¼ hours (or 6¼ hours in a slow cooker)

1 tablespoon olive oil
1 onion, chopped
1 garlic clove, crushed
2 green chilies, seeded and chopped
1 teaspoon ground coriander
1 teaspoon ground cumin
½ teaspoon chili powder

2 teaspoons garam masala
2 teaspoons curry powder
14oz (2¾ cups) cubed skinless chicken breast
2 tablespoons all-purpose flour
olive oil spray
2¼ cups tomato sauce
sea salt and freshly ground black pepper
Herbed Cauliflower Pilaf (see page 327), to serve (optional)

1 Preheat the oven to 325°F, or set the slow cooker to Low. Heat the oil in a nonstick skillet over medium heat, and fry the onion for 5 minutes until soft. Add the garlic, chilies and spices, and fry for another 1 minute (add a splash of water if the mixture sticks to the pan).
2 Transfer to a casserole or the slow cooker. Put the chicken in a bowl and add the flour. Season with salt and pepper and stir to coat the chicken. Spray the skillet with oil spray and fry the chicken for 4–5 minutes until browned. Add a splash of water and stir to deglaze the pan, scraping up any sticky juices to coat the chicken. Stir in the tomao sauce and bring to a boil.
3 Transfer the mixture to the casserole or slow cooker. Stir and cover, then put the casserole in the oven and cook for 2 hours, or cook in the slow cooker for 6 hours or until tender. If the mixture in the casserole becomes too dry, add a little more water. There will be plenty for the slow cooker as less water evaporates. Serve with Herbed Cauliflower Pilaf.

Nutritional information per serving
Kcals **231** Protein **26g** Carbohydrate **16g** Fat **4g**

Best for Tired Hunger. Lack of sleep leads to increased appetite, but the vitamin C in tomatoes makes the sleep hormone melatonin. Also good for 🥛 ❄️

Pork and Thyme Casserole

This really is a one-pot dish, as you have protein from the pork, and good carbs and plenty of fiber from the vegetables, barley and split peas.

Serves: 4
Preparation time: 15 minutes
Cooking time: 2½ hours (or 6½ hours in a slow cooker)

olive oil spray
1 onion, chopped
4 garlic cloves, crushed
4 carrots, peeled and cut into thick chunks
1lb pork tenderloin, cut into chunks

2½ cups chicken bouillon
¼ cup pearl barley
¼ cup split peas
leaves from 2 thyme sprigs
4 bay leaves
⅓ cup frozen peas, defrosted
sea salt and freshly ground black pepper

1 Preheat the oven to 325°F, or set the slow cooker to Low. Put a nonstick skillet over medium heat and spray with oil, then fry the onion for 5 minutes until soft. Add the garlic and carrots, and fry for 1 minute (add a splash of water if the mixture sticks to the pan).
2 Transfer to a large casserole or the slow cooker. Spray the skillet with oil and gently fry the pork for 4–5 minutes to brown. Add a splash of water and stir to deglaze the pan, scraping up any sticky juices to coat the pork.
3 Transfer to the casserole or slow cooker and add the remaining ingredients, except the frozen peas. Season with salt and pepper. Stir and cover, then put the casserole in the oven and cook for 2 hours, or cook in the slow cooker for 4–6 hours. Stir in the peas and cook for another 15 minutes, then serve.

Nutritional information per serving
Kcals **279** Protein **63g** Carbohydrate **37g** Fat **10g**

Best for Never-Full Hunger. Barley is a low-GI whole grain that releases its sugar slowly, thus keeping blood sugar and mood stable. Its high fiber content also means that you feel fuller for longer. Also good for 🍲 🍲

Feel-Good Chili

Why feel-good? Because turkey is much higher in tryptophan—the amino acid you need to make the feel-good hormone serotonin—than beef.

Serves: 4
Preparation time: 15 minutes
Cooking time: 2¾ hours (or 8¼ hours in a slow cooker)

1 tablespoon olive oil
1 onion, chopped
1 teaspoon ground cumin
1 teaspoon smoked paprika
1 carrot, peeled and chopped
1 leek, chopped
1 red bell pepper, seeded and chopped
1 yellow bell pepper, seeded and chopped

2 red chilies, seeded and finely sliced
olive oil spray
1 lb ground turkey
3 x 14oz cans chopped tomatoes
2 teaspoons Worcestershire sauce
1 x 14oz can red kidney beans, drained and rinsed
1 bunch of fresh cilantro, leaves chopped
juice of 2 limes
sea salt and freshly ground black pepper
4 tablespoons fat-free Greek yogurt, to serve

1 Preheat the oven to 325°F, or set the slow cooker to Low. Heat the oil in a nonstick skillet over medium heat, and fry the onion for 3–4 minutes to soften. Add the spices and fry for 1 minute (add a splash of water if the mixture sticks to the pan). Stir in the carrot, leek, bell peppers and chilies. Transfer to a casserole or the slow cooker.
2 Spray the skillet with oil and add the turkey. Stir-fry for 5–7 minutes to brown, then transfer to the casserole or slow cooker. Add the remaining ingredients except the lime juice. Season with salt and pepper. Stir and cover, then put the casserole in the oven and cook for 2½ hours, or cook in the slow cooker for 6–8 hours. Stir in the lime juice and serve with yogurt.

Nutritional information per serving
Kcals **376** Protein **37g** Carbohydrate **46g** Fat **11g**

Best for Emotional Hunger. The abundance of vitamin C in bell peppers can support the adrenal glands, to help us deal with stress and emotional eating. Also good for

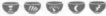

Cajun Spiced Trout

Trout is a good substitute for salmon with the same healthy oils.

Serves: 2
Preparation time: 10 minutes
Cooking time: 10 minutes

1 teaspoon cumin seeds
1 teaspoon coriander seeds
1 teaspoon paprika
1 teaspoon ground cinnamon
1 teaspoon cayenne pepper
2 trout fillets, 4¼oz each,
   skin on
1 tablespoon olive oil
juice of 1 lemon

For the tomato sauce
1 x 14oz can chopped tomatoes
4 tablespoons basil leaves
1 teaspoon stevia-based granulated
   sweetener
a pinch of sea salt

For the zucchini salad
2 zucchinis
juice of 1 lemon
sea salt and freshly ground black
   pepper

1 Preheat the oven to 400°F. Put the cumin and coriander seeds in a mortar and grind to a smooth powder using a pestle. Mix in the remaining spices, then rub this into the trout and set aside.
2 To make the tomato sauce, put all the ingredients into a blender or food processor and blend until smooth. Pour into a saucepan over medium heat and heat gently for 3 minutes, without boiling.
3 Heat the oil in an ovenproof skillet over medium heat. Add the trout, skin-side down, and cook for 1 minute, then cook the other side for 1 minute. Add the lemon juice and transfer the pan to the oven to bake for 3 minutes.
4 To make the zucchini salad, use a vegetable peeler to slice the zucchini into ribbons. Put them in a bowl and add the lemon juice. Season with salt and pepper. Serve the trout drizzled with sauce, with the zucchini salad.

Nutritional information per serving
Kcals **343** Protein **28g** Carbohydrate **9g** Fat **9g**

Best for Cravings Hunger. Cinnamon is well researched as an aid to good blood sugar balance. Stable blood sugar evens out mood and prevents bingeing and comfort eating. Also good for

Tuna Steak with Fava Beans, Snow Peas and Oregano Oil

Flavored oils are a clever way to make a quick and intensely flavored sauce, as long as you exercise some self-control. Oregano oil is my favorite.

Serves: 2
Preparation time: 10 minutes
Cooking time: 10 minutes

olive oil spray
1 small bunch of oregano leaves
a pinch of sea sea salt
juice of 1 lemon

2 tablespoons extra-virgin olive oil
2 cups frozen fava beans, defrosted
2½ cups fresh snow peas
1 tablespoon chopped mint leaves
2 fresh tuna steaks, 4¼oz each
sea salt and freshly ground black
   pepper

1 Put a griddle pan over medium-high heat and spray with oil. Put the oregano in a mortar and add the salt, lemon juice and olive oil. Pound with a pestle until combined, then set aside.
2 Put the fava beans and snow peas in a steamer over boiling water and cook for 3–4 minutes or until just tender. Stir in the mint. Drain the pan and set aside.
3 Meanwhile, season the tuna and put it on the griddle pan. Cook for 2–3 minutes on each side until cooked through. Serve the tuna on top of the snow peas and beans, and drizzle with the oregano oil.

Nutritional information per serving
Kcals **415** Protein **43g** Carbohydrate **17g** Fat **17g**

Best for 40+ Hunger. Fava beans are high in fiber, which helps the body excrete toxic substances such as "old" hormones. This can improve hormone balance and reduce PMS overeating and estrogen-driven weight gain in 40+ men and women. Also good for 🥗 🥗 🥗 🥗 🌙

Spaghetti with Charbroiled Squid and Caponata

....

Don't get overexcited. The serving size of spaghetti isn't huge. But if you love pasta, here it is, with the Italian eggplant dish of caponata. Get the squid cleaned at the fish counter or buy it frozen, already cut into rings— very easy.

Serves: 2
Preparation time: 15 minutes
Cooking time: 20 minutes

olive oil spray
1 onion, chopped
2 celery stalks, chopped
2 garlic cloves, crushed
1½ heaping cups cherry tomatoes
1 eggplant, cut into ½-inch dice

1 teaspoon stevia-based granulated
  sweetener
1 tablespoon balsamic vinegar
1 tablespoon capers, rinsed
6 pitted black olives, chopped
3½oz whole-wheat spaghetti
9oz squid rings
sea salt and freshly ground black
  pepper

1 Put a griddle pan over medium-high heat. Meanwhile, put a nonstick saucepan over medium heat and spray with oil, then fry the onion for 5 minutes or until soft. Add the celery and garlic, and fry for 1 minute, then add the tomatoes and eggplant. Fry for 3–4 minutes until the tomatoes start to collapse. Add the sweetener, vinegar, capers and olives, and fry for 2–3 minutes (add a splash of water if the mixture sticks to the pan).
2 Meanwhile, bring a large saucepan of salted water to a boil over high heat. Add the spaghetti and cook for 8–10 minutes, or according to the package instructions, until tender with a bite in the center. Drain and set aside.
3 Season the squid with pepper and cook on the griddle for 2–3 minutes on each side until cooked through and charred around the edges. Serve the caponata over the spaghetti with the squid rings on top.

Nutritional information per serving
Kcals **391** Protein **87g** Carbohydrate **83g** Fat **3g**

Best for Tired Hunger, because squid contains zinc, which supports the energy-boosting thyroid gland. Also good for 🥣 🥣 🥣 🥣

Tofu Mutter Paneer with Chapatis

Most Indian breads contain ghee (fried butter). Chapatis are the exception.
They are made with whole-wheat flour and are fat-free and easy to make.

Serves: 2
Preparation time: 20 minutes
Cooking time: 25 minutes

¾ cup whole-wheat flour, plus extra
    for dusting
olive oil spray
1 teaspoon mustard seeds
1 teaspoon cumin seeds
1 small onion, chopped

1 tomato, chopped
1 teaspoon tomato paste
½ teaspoon ground cumin
½ teaspoon ground coriander
a pinch of chili powder
a pinch of ground turmeric
7oz firm tofu, drained and cube
2¼ cups frozen peas
1 tablespoon chopped cilantro leaves

1 Put the flour in a bowl and gradually add ¼ cup cold water, while using your
hands to mix the water to make a soft, elastic dough. Knead the dough on a
lightly floured work suface for 3–4 minutes.

2 Divide the dough into two balls, flatten them, then use a rolling pin to roll
out the dough to 6-inch discs. Heat a dry nonstick skillet over medium heat.
Add a disc and cook for 30 seconds or until it starts to bubble, then flip it
over to cook the other side. Put on a plate and cover with a clean dish towel
to keep warm. Repeat with the other disc.

3 To make the curry, put a large nonstick saucepan over medium heat and
spray with oil. Fry the mustard and cumin seeds until the mustard starts to
pop. Add the onion and cook for 4 minutes or until softened (add a splash
of water if the mixture sticks to the pan). Add the tomato, tomato paste and
ground spices. Simmer for 5 minutes, then add the tofu and a scant ⅓ cup
water. Bring to a boil and add the peas, then simmer for 10 minutes. Add the
cilantro and serve the curry with the chapatis.

> **Nutritional information per serving**
> Kcals **467** Protein **17g** Carbohydrate **21g** Fat **12g**

 Best for Emotional Hunger. Peas contain high levels
of vitamin C. This is essential to help us make the
appetite-suppressant hormone serotonin. Also good
for 🍽 💤 40+

Greek Vegetable and Halloumi Stew

Halloumi is a Greek, or more usually Cypriot, cheese made from sheep's milk. This makes it easier on the stomach for those with a dairy intolerance. It's also one of the lower-fat cheeses.

Serves: 4
Preparation time: 15 minutes
Cooking time: 1 hour 10 minutes (or 3 hours 10 minutes in a slow cooker)

1 tablespoon olive oil
1 red onion, chopped
3 garlic cloves, crushed
1 small red chili, seeded and chopped

2 zucchinis, sliced
3 x 14oz cans chopped tomatoes
1 eggplant, sliced
2½ cups vegetable bouillon
1 bay leaf
olive oil spray
10½oz halloumi cheese, sliced
sea salt and freshly ground black pepper

1 Preheat the oven to 325°F, or set the slow cooker to Low.
Heat the oil in a nonstick saucepan over medium heat, then fry the onion for 5 minutes or until soft. Add the garlic and fry for 1 minute (add a splash of water if the mixture sticks to the pan).
2 Transfer to a large casserole or the slow cooker and add the remaining ingredients, except the oil spray and halloumi cheese. Season with salt and pepper. Stir and cover, then put the casserole in the oven and cook for 1 hour, or cook in the slow cooker for 3 hours.
3 Ten minutes before serving, put a griddle pan over medium-high heat and spray with oil. Griddle the halloumi slices until golden, turning once. Serve the stew topped with the halloumi slices.

Nutritional information per serving
Kcals **336** Protein **19g** Carbohydrate **13g** Fat **20g**

Best for Hedonistic Hunger. Dieters used to be told to avoid cheese, but the calcium in cheese is now believed to switch off the hunger hormone ghrelin. Also good for

Mushroom and Lentil Stew with Tofu

Far removed from those stereotypical brown vegan mushes, this tastes great, and by adding the tofu you kick it up a notch protein-wise.

Serves: 4
Preparation time: 20 minutes, plus 10 minutes soaking
Cooking time: 2 hours 10 minutes (or 5 hours 10 minutes in a slow cooker)

1 cup dried shiitake mushrooms
1 teaspoon olive oil
1 onion, finely chopped
1 garlic clove, crushed
3 cups button mushrooms

8½ cups vegetable bouillon, as needed
heaping ¾ cup pearl barley
heaping ¾ cup red lentils
1 teaspoon dried mixed herbs
2 bay leaves
1 teaspoon dried basil
14oz firm tofu, drained and cut into cubes
sea salt and freshly ground black pepper

1 Preheat the oven to 325°F, or set the slow cooker to Low. Put the shiitake mushrooms in a bowl and pour over boiling water to cover. Leave to soak for 10 minutes.

2 Heat the oil in a nonstick saucepan over medium heat, and fry the onion for 5 minutes until soft. Remove the shiitake from the soaking liquid and snip out the stalks using scissors. Discard the stalks. Strain the liquid through a fine strainer into a measuring cup. Chop the shiitake caps and add to the pan, followed by the garlic and button mushrooms. Fry for 1 minute (add a splash of the soaking liquid if the mixture sticks to the pan). Make up the remaining soaking liquid to 8½ cups with the vegetable bouillon.

3 Pour the liquid into a large casserole or slow cooker and add all the remaining ingredients. Season, stir and cover, then put the casserole in the oven and cook for 2 hours, or cook in the slow cooker for 5 hours. Serve.

> **Nutritional information per serving**
> Kcals **288** Protein **20g** Carbohydrate **38g** Fat **15g**

Best for PMS Hunger. The zinc in mushrooms supports thyroid function, speeding up your metabolism. It also makes the appetite-suppressant serotonin, which can be low premenstrually. Also good for 🥣 🥣 🥣 🥣 🥣

Persian Chicken Skewers with Herbed Cauliflower Pilaf

....

This is a substantial dinner, and the dates give it a really lovely sweetness.

Serves: 4
Preparation time: 15 minutes
Cooking time: 10 minutes

olive oil spray
1lb skinless chicken breast, cubed
1 large zucchini, cut into chunks
8 pitted dried dates, cut into quarters
2 tablespoons soy sauce
2 tablespoons agave syrup
2 tablespoons sesame seeds

For the herbed cauliflower pilaf
½ medium cauliflower, roughly
   chopped
zest and juice of 2 lemons
1 large handful of parsley, leaves
   chopped
1 large handful of mint, leaves
   chopped
1 large handful of basil, leaves
   chopped
sea salt and freshly ground black
   pepper

1 Soak four wooden skewers in a bowl of cold water. Meanwhile, put the cauliflower for the pilaf into a food processor and process until the consistency of rice. Tip into a bowl and set aside. Put a griddle pan over medium-high heat and spray with oil.
2 Thread the chicken, zucchini and dates alternately onto the skewers. Put the soy sauce, agave syrup and sesame seeds in a bowl and mix together, then use a pastry brush to brush over the skewered ingredients. Cook on the griddle for 5–7 minutes, turning and basting until all the sides are cooked.
3 Meanwhile, put the cauliflower in a steamer over boiling water for 3 minutes, or in the microwave on full power for 2 minutes. Stir in the lemon zest and juice, and the herbs. Season with salt and pepper. Heat the remaining dressing in a pan until boiling. Serve the pilaf with the skewers on top and drizzle over the dressing.

Nutritional information per serving
Kcals **372** Protein **33g** Carbohydrate **47g** Fat **5g**

Best for PMS Hunger. Parsley is a diuretic. This means it helps the body rid itself of excess water, so it can reduce bloating. Also good for 🥣 🥣 🥣 🥣

Venison with Dukkah Rub and Quinoa Salad

Lean venison is also free-range and contains healthy omega-3 fats.

Serves: 4
Preparation time: 15 minutes
Cooking time: 25 minutes, plus cooling

1 teaspoon cloves
1 teaspoon fennel seeds
1 teaspoon coriander seeds
1 teaspoon cumin seeds
a pinch of ground turmeric
a pinch of chili powder
heaping ¼ cup pistachio nuts, chopped
2 tablespoons agave syrup
juice of 1 orange

2 tablespoons olive oil
4 venison steaks, 3½oz each
olive oil spray

For the quinoa salad
¾ cup quinoa
1 tablespoon chopped mint leaves
1 tablespoon chopped parsley leaves
1 red bell pepper, seeded and finely sliced
1 cucumber, diced
1 red onion, diced
juice of 1 lemon
sea salt and freshly ground black pepper

1 To make the quinoa salad, put the quinoa in a saucepan over high heat with twice the volume of water and a pinch of salt. Bring to a boil, then cover and simmer for 10–15 minutes until the quinoa has absorbed all the water. Set aside and, when slightly cooler, stir in the remaining salad ingredients. Season with salt and pepper.

2 Put the spices in a nonstick skillet over medium heat and dry-fry until they release their aroma. Grind using a mortar and pestle. Transfer to a bowl and add the nuts, agave syrup, orange juice and olive oil. Mix together, then use to rub over the steaks. Put a griddle pan over high heat and spray with oil. Griddle the steaks for 2–3 minutes on each side. Serve with the salad.

Nutritional information per serving
Kcals **476** Protein **30g** Carbohydrate **35g** Fat **23g**

Best for Cravings Hunger. Quinoa contains complete protein—that is, the full range of amino acids to build healthy tissues. It also has a low GI, so it keeps blood sugar stable, reducing cravings. Also good for 🍲 🍴 🍲

Boeuf Bourguignon with Broccoli Mash

A real French classic.

Serves: 4
Preparation time: 20 minutes
Cooking time: 3¼ hours (or 8¼ hours in a slow cooker)

1 tablespoon olive oil
1 onion, chopped
2 garlic cloves, crushed
3 cups button mushrooms
2½ cups carrots, peeled and chopped

olive oil spray
14oz lean braising steak, cubed
1 tablespoon whole-wheat flour
scant 1⅓ cups red wine
1 bouquet garni
14oz broccoli, roughly chopped
juice of ½ lemon
2½ cups sugar snap peas
sea salt and freshly ground black pepper

1 Preheat the oven to 325°F, or set the slow cooker to Low.
Heat the oil in a nonstick skillet over medium heat, then fry the onion for 5 minutes or until soft. Add the garlic, mushrooms and carrots, and fry for 1 minute (add a splash of water if the mixture sticks to the pan). Transfer to a casserole or the slow cooker. Spray the skillet with oil. Toss the beef in the flour and gently fry for 4–5 minutes to brown all over, adding more oil if needed. Add a splash of the wine and stir to deglaze the pan.
2 Transfer to the casserole or slow cooker and add the remaining wine and the bouquet garni. Season, stir and cover, then cook the casserole in the oven for 2–3 hours, or cook in the slow cooker for 6–8 hours until tender. Meanwhile, put the broccoli in a steamer over boiling water and cook for 12 minutes or until tender. Transfer to a blender or food processor and add the lemon juice. Season with pepper and blend to a purée. Steam the peas for 4 minutes or until crisp-tender. Serve the beef with the broccoli and peas.

Nutritional information per serving
Kcals **455** Protein **74g** Carbohydrate **32g** Fat **27g**

Best for Tired Hunger. Beef is packed full of energy-boosting iron, so it could reduce tired hunger. Also good for

Salt-Crusted Sea Bass with Avocado and Zucchini Salad

Bake the fish in a salt crust, then use a knife to break the crust at the table.

Serves: 4
Preparation time: 20 minutes
Cooking time: 35 minutes

1 bunch of thyme
1 sea bass, about 1lb 2oz, or
   2 smaller sea bass, about 9oz each,
   head on but cleaned
4 egg whites
300g/10½oz coarse sea salt
4 zucchinis
1⅓ cups frozen fava beans, defrosted
4 tablespoons chopped parsley leaves

2 shallots, sliced into rings
2 little gem lettuces, leaves separated
1 avocado, peeled, pitted and thinly
   sliced

For the dressing
1 teaspoon English mustard
1 tablespoon red wine vinegar
a squeeze of lemon juice
2 tablespoons olive oil
a pinch of stevia-based granulated
   sweetener

1 Preheat the oven to 400°F. Put the thyme inside the fish. Whisk the egg whites in a clean bowl until they form soft peaks. Fold in the salt. Line a baking sheet with parchment paper and spread one-third of the mixture over it. Lay the bass on top and spread over the remaining salt mix.
2 Bake the fish for 30–35 minutes (or 25 minutes for smaller fish). Meanwhile, use a vegetable peeler to slice the zucchini into ribbons. Put the fava beans in a steamer over boiling water and cook for 3 minutes. Add the zucchini for 1 minute more, drain in a colander and refresh under cold water. Drain, then pat dry with paper towels. Tip into a bowl and add the parsley, shallots and lettuce. Mix the dressing in a bowl, then add to the salad and toss. Add the avocado and serve with the bass.

Nutritional information per serving
Kcals **357** Protein **33g** Carbohydrate **11g** Fat **22g**

Best for Emotional Hunger. Sea bass is one of the lesser-known oily fish. As such, it is a good source of omega-3 fats, and these have been shown to fight depression, which can lead to overeating. Also good for

Mini Fish Pies with Oaty Crumble Topping

There are no desserts in this book (whaaaat!), so this is the closest you'll get to an apple crumble. It's savory, obviously, but still pretty comforting.

Serves: 4
Preparation time: 20 minutes, plus cooling
Cooking time: 35 minutes
1½lb baby spinach leaves
olive oil spray
2 onions, chopped
2 garlic cloves, crushed
2 x 14oz cans chopped tomatoes
1 teaspoon stevia-based granulated sweetener
1lb white fish fillet, skinned and cut into pieces
1 bunch of basil, leaves shredded
3 tablespoons fresh whole-wheat bread crumbs
4 tablespoons freshly grated Parmesan cheese
4 tablespoons rolled oats
sea salt and freshly ground black pepper
mixed green salad, to serve

1 Preheat the oven to 350°F. Put the spinach in a colander over the sink and pour boiling water over to wilt it (you may have to do this in batches). Leave to cool, then squeeze out the liquid. Season it with salt and pepper, then set aside. Put a nonstick saucepan over medium heat and spray with oil, then fry the onions for 5 minutes or until soft. Add the garlic and fry for 1 minute (add a splash of water if the mixture sticks to the pan). Add the tomatoes and sweetener and bring to a boil, then reduce the heat and simmer for 5 minutes to reduce by one-third. Add the fish and cook for 2 minutes. Take the pan off the heat and add the basil.
2 Put a spoonful of tomato sauce into the base of two individual ramekins or ovenproof dishes, then add the spinach, the fish and the remaining sauce.
3 In a bowl, mix together the bread crumbs, Parmesan and oats. Season with salt and pepper, then sprinkle the mixture over the top of the sauce. Cook in the oven for 20 minutes or until the tops are golden. Serve with a green salad.

Nutritional information per serving
Kcals **341** Protein **33g** Carbohydrate **31g** Fat **6g**

 Best for Cravings Hunger. Oats contain the amino acid tyrosine – the chemical precursor for the anti-craving hormone dopamine. Also good for

Japanese Marinated Tofu with Soba Noodles

Tofu always tastes better if you marinate it, so take the time to do this in the morning so that it's ready to cook in the evening. Soba noodles (made from buckwheat) are better than brown noodles, because they are lower in carbs.

Serves: 4
Preparation time: 10 minutes, plus 4 hours marinating
Cooking time: 15 minutes

1lb firm tofu, drained and cubed
7oz soba noodles
14oz sugar snap peas

For the Japanese marinade
2 tablespoons sesame oil
zest and juice of 2 limes
2 teaspoons dried chili flakes
½ cup soy sauce
1 tablespoon agave syrup

1 Put the marinade ingredients in a bowl and mix together well. Add the tofu and stir gently to coat. Cover and chill for at least 4 hours.
2 Bring a large saucepan of water to a boil over high heat. Add the noodles and cook for 10–12 minutes, or according to the package instructions, until tender. Add the sugar snap peas for the last 4 minutes. Drain and set aside.
3 Meanwhile, heat a wok over medium-high heat and carefully pour in the tofu and its marinade. Cover the wok and simmer for 2 minutes. Serve the noodles and sugar snap peas topped with the tofu.

Nutritional information per serving
Kcals 367 Protein 41g Carbohydrate 40g Fat 28g

Best for 40+ Hunger. Buckwheat is high in essential fats, which can improve cell sensitivity and reduce hormonally driven fat storage, especially important for 40+ Hunger.
Also good for 🥣 🥣 🥣

Roasted Vegetables with Broccoli and Pomegranate Couscous

My healthy broccoli "couscous" looks pretty with the pomegranate seeds.

Serves: 4
Preparation time: 15 minutes
Cooking time: 30 minutes

olive oil spray
4 carrots, peeled and cut into chunks
4 parsnips, cut into chunks
4 red onions, cut into quarters
4 red bell peppers, seeded and cut into chunks
2 tablespoons olive oil
1 teaspoon ground cumin
1 teaspoon paprika
1 teaspoon ground cinnamon
1 teaspoon chili powder

1 x 14oz can chopped tomatoes
heaping ⅓ cup chopped dried apricots
2 teaspoons agave syrup
7oz feta cheese, crumbled
sea salt and freshly ground black pepper

For the broccoli couscous
1 large bunch broccoli, chopped
1 large handful of mint leaves
1 large handful of parsley leaves
juice of 1 orange
2 tablespoons balsamic vinegar
seeds from 1 pomegranate

1 Preheat the oven to 400°F. Spray a roasting pan with oil, then add the vegetables. Spray with oil, season and roast for 20–30 minutes until starting to brown. Heat the olive oil in a large nonstick skillet over medium heat and fry the spices for 1 minute. Add the tomatoes, apricots and agave syrup. Bring to a boil, then simmer for 5 minutes or until the sauce reduces slightly. Add the roasted vegetables and set aside.

2 To make the couscous, put the broccoli and herbs in a food processor and process until the consistency of rice. Mix the orange juice and vinegar in a bowl, then stir into the broccoli and add the pomegranate seeds. Season with salt and pepper, then serve the couscous with the vegetables and the feta.

Nutritional information per serving
Kcals **415** Protein **22g** Carbohydrate **47g** Fat **4g**

Best for PMS Hunger. Dried fruit, such as apricots, is high in energy-giving iron, providing you with the oomph to exercise. Also good for 🥣 🥣 🥣 🥣 🥣 🥣

Index

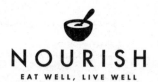

NOURISH
EAT WELL, LIVE WELL

Here at Nourish we're all about wellbeing through food
and drink – irresistible dishes with a serious good-for-you factor.
If you want to eat and drink delicious things that set you up for the
day, suit any special diets, keep you healthy and make the most
of the ingredients you have, we've got some great ideas to share
with you. Come over to our blog for wholesome recipes and fresh
inspiration – nourishbooks.com